THE
STARCH
BLOCKER
DIET

THE STARCH BLOCKER DIET

Steven Rosenblatt, M.D., Ph.D.,
and Cameron Stauth

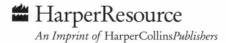 HarperResource

An Imprint of HarperCollins*Publishers*

HarperCollins books may be purchased for educational, business, or sales promotional use. For information, please write: Special Markets Department, HarperCollins Publishers Inc., 10 East 53rd Street, New York, NY 10022.

FIRST EDITION

Designed by Nancy Singer Olaguera

Library of Congress Cataloging-in-Publication Data has been applied for.

ISBN 0-06-054823-1

03 04 05 06 07 ❖/RRD 10 9 8 7 6 5 4 3 2 1

For my "sisters," Faith Baynes and Jaque Nutt.
                                            —Cameron Stauth

For my children: May you live your lives with passion and joy.
                                            —Steven Rosenblatt

CONTENTS

ACKNOWLEDGMENTS

The authors appreciate very much the effort and energy of the following people, who made important contributions to this book. Thanks!

To Toni Sciarra, for sculpting the book—making changes both sweeping and minute—and for having the vision to recognize the good this book could bring to people.

To Richard Pine, for making the uncertain profession of writing somehow seem secure.

To Sandra Stahl, for turning ideas into pages.

To David Shaw, for providing the spark that ignited the project.

To Herman H. Rappaport, for guidance and support.

To Philippe and Susan Boulot, world-class chefs, who brought artistry to a book about science.

To Mitch Skop, for bringing starch blockers to the American people.

And to Lorraine and Vernon Stauth, who did their work on this book in what seems like another lifetime, now brought back.

Final billing and great gratitude goes to Chris Ade, director of research for the book, who found order in chaos, separated science from fiction, and brought good cheer every day to a difficult and demanding task.

INTRODUCTION

by Jay Udani, M.D.
Medical Director, Integrative Medicine Program
Northridge Hospital Medical Center

America's epidemic of obesity must be ended, and it is my carefully considered opinion, based upon my own clinical research, that the substance known as starch blockers represents one of the best weapons we now have in the war against obesity.

At present, the epidemic is increasing at a stunning pace. Estimates vary, but obesity is widely believed to have doubled between the late 1970s and the early 1990s, and has increased at an even faster rate since then. Since 1980, childhood obesity has tripled.

Now more than half of all Americans are either overweight or obese, and even an estimated 25% of American children are overweight, and about 15% are obese.

The consequences are horrendous. Diabetes incidence is at an all-time high, and it is increasingly common among children. Other weight-related diseases are among our current most common causes of debilitation and death, including coronary artery disease, hypertension, degenerative arthritis, and obstructive sleep apnea. These diseases, combined with diabetes, account for about 300,000 deaths annually.

Overweight and obesity also contribute significantly, through secondary causative factors, to increased risk of infection, incidence of certain cancers, and major depression.

This constellation of diseases, revolving around simple caloric excess, represents the greatest single threat to the long-range health of the American public. In the very near future, caloric excess will surpass even smoking as America's deadliest public health risk factor.

For many years, the medical profession has struggled to treat obesity with various diets, but this effort has thus far failed. No existing diet has been shown to reverse obesity or overweight in large groups of people over extended periods of time. Most people just can't seem to stay on weight control diets. Compliance with low-calorie and low-fat diets has been quite poor in virtually all long-term studies. Extended compliance has also been poor among diets that are intended to influence the metabolism, such as low-carbohydrate diets. Most people do not feel sufficiently comfortable on restrictive diets to maintain them over periods of months or years.

There are, of course, exceptions to this general rule. Some people do succeed, just as a relatively small percentage of people who try to stop smoking succeed. However, long-term success on weight loss diets occurs even less often than long-term abstinence from smoking. The average rate of success for weight control diets is approximately 10%.

The medical and pharmaceutical professions have also tried to devise medications that will solve the dilemma of obesity, applying several different classes of drugs. One class consists of medications that increase the activity of the neurotransmitter serotonin, which enhances satiety. Another approach has involved the use of stimulating noradrenergic agents, which also enhance satiety, as well as increase energy. In addition, pharmaceutical drugs have been created that interfere with the digestion of fat and starch.

None of these diet drugs has achieved widespread use. In addition, they all have side effects. For example, the most popular of the serotonin-enhancing agents, commonly called "Fen-Phen," created serious heart and lung problems, even with very minimal use. Similarly, the pharmaceutical drugs that interfere with fat and starch digestion also created significant negative consequences, such as severe bloating, fecal incontinence, and the loss of fat-soluble vitamins.

Again, there have been exceptions among patients to this pattern of failure. Unfortunately, though, the exceptions have been too few and far between.

Over these years of struggle and failure, it has become apparent that weight management requires an approach that is safe, very powerful, and compatible with long-term use. It has been exceedingly difficult to find a substance that provides this rare combination of factors.

Finally, though, there is reason for great optimism. After more than thirty years of research, development, and testing, the strategy of starch calorie neutralization, employing a substance known as Phase 2 fulfulls the demand for an approach to weight management that appears to be safe, very powerful, and appropriate for long-term use.

The story of Phase 2 began in the 1970s, when scientists first described an apparent "antinutrient" that somehow caused weight loss in animals. The most recent chapter of this story unfolded in my own medical facility, when a clinical study that I directed showed that Phase 2, which blocks starch calorie digestion created a positive trend in weight loss. More importantly, the participants were not compelled to eat a calorie-resticted diet or to exercise.

In my study, the patients who took Phase 2 averaged a degree of weight loss that was 230% greater than that of patients taking placebos. They also successfully lost an average of one and one-half inches around their waists in eight weeks.

Most intriguing of all, the volunteers who took Phase 2 *felt* much better than those on placebos, which is the opposite of the usual response among people who are losing weight. Typically, people on weight loss diets experience increased hunger and irritability, and decreased energy. In my study, though, the subjects on Phase 2 showed improvements in their energy levels, even though Phase 2 is not a stimulant.

This improvement in how people felt is of paramount importance. The primary reason most people can't lose weight and keep it off is simply that they don't feel good on conventional, restrictive diets. Conventional diets do not just deprive people psychologically, but also physiologically. Restrictive diets just don't supply enough nutrients and bulk to keep people from becoming hungry.

Thus, Phase 2 presents a new paradigm in modern weight management. It allows people to eat normal foods in normal amounts. It is not a stimulant. Safety data to date indicates that it appears to be appropriate for long-term use. And it makes people feel better, instead of worse.

Therefore, Phase 2 apparantly offers a viable approach to the modern epidemic of overweight and obesity.

This book, by two of the leading experts on the science and application of starch calorie neutralization, is an invaluable source of information about this medical advance. Dr. Steven Rosenblatt was among the first clinicians ever to embrace the clinical application of this approach, and Cameron Stauth was the first medical author ever to report on this breakthrough, more than twenty years ago. Together, they bring a wealth of experience and expertise to an extremely important topic. They tell people how to use Phase 2 as part of a balanced, integrated program that maximizes the benefit of this exciting new strategy in weight management. They demonstrate that participating in their comprehensive three-step program is far more valuable for people than just taking Phase 2, and hoping for the best.

The program will not end America's epidemic of obesity overnight. This epidemic can be ended only by the American people themselves. Bringing this information to their attention, though, may one day be seen as the first major step that was taken in helping to restore the battered health of the people of this country.

Dr. Jay Udani is a former chief resident of internal medicine at Cedars-Sinai Medical Center, a Harvard Medical School research fellow, a contributor to the *Journal of the American Medical Association,* and director of the Integrative Medicine Program at Northridge Hospital, and is a UCLA Clinical Instructor.

PART ONE

THE STARCH BLOCKER STRATEGY

ONE

BEYOND DENIAL DIETS

Finally: A Sane Solution to the Low-Carb Revolution

I was facing the kind of day that would once have broken my heart. I was scheduled to see three patients who all had the same problem, one that medical science has long struggled unsuccessfully to solve. As recently as a year ago, a day like this would have left me in despair.

My greatest source of pain as a doctor—the greatest pain of almost all doctors—is *knowing* the solution to a problem but being unable to act on it. My three patients had a problem that has always been one of those frustrating, intractable conditions that seems as if it should be solvable, but usually isn't: weight control.

For many years, I have known the answer. Virtually everyone knows it: Eat fewer calories. But how do you *achieve* this, in the real world, with real people, day after day, year after year? That is the question that no doctor, until recently, has been able to adequately answer.

Sure, there are dozens of aggressive low-calorie, low-carbohydrate, low-fat diets, some of them quite capable of inducing weight loss—*if* people can stay on them. But who can? Apparently, not many of us, since obesity has doubled in the past twenty years, and morbid obesity has quadrupled, with most of that increase coming in just the last decade. About 33% of all American people are currently obese, and 61% are at least overweight. Even 40% of children are overweight or obese. That's 150 million people—a horrifying public health catastrophe.

All of the existing diets that have failed to stop this epidemic have different advantages. Some more effectively provide sufficient nutrients, and others are better at keeping the cardiovascular system free of fats. A few excel at controlling key metabolic factors, such as insulin output. However, they all run headlong into the same oppressive problem: *hunger.*

Hunger overcomes the weight management motivations of even extremely strong-willed people. It's an almost irresistible primal force that people have been programmed over the course of a million years of evolution to hate—even to fear. It's a relentless emptiness that strikes not just the body but also the brain, which requires 25% of all calories consumed by adults, and up to 50% of all calories consumed by children. Hunger whispers a primeval message to the brain and the body that starvation is lurking, and that eating is absolutely necessary *now.* It makes people feel weak, ravenous, irritable—and desperate.

Physical hunger is a terribly invasive force, but it's not the only kind of hunger that dieters have long been unable to endure. There is also a strong psychological aspect to hunger. We are not only neurologically programmed to hate and fear hunger, but we are also conditioned by evolutionary forces to crave and appreciate the exquisite tastes of various foods, and to desire these foods as a central part of our enjoyment of life.

Food, after all, is far more than just calories.

Food is, in fact, the veritable essence and elixir of life—the sustaining, nurturing product of our earth, air, sun, and water. It is simply human nature to desire it.

Thus, there is a missing element in virtually all current weight control diets, which are effective *only when desired foods are denied.* That element is the *human element.*

If human beings were machines, weight control would be easy. We would all simply consume the exact number of calories we need, and then flip a switch to turn consumption off. But we're not machines. We are finite beings, full of feelings, destined eventually to die, but determined to live a little first, and to savor the joys of our senses during our stay on this earth.

Thus, human nature itself is the primary reason 90% of all weight loss diets fail. People just can't—or won't—hold out indefinitely against the physical and psychological onslaught of hunger.

So they eat.

Throughout almost all of our million-year human history, this natural desire to eat a rich and varied diet caused only occasional problems, because the vast majority of people were very physically active. As recently as the early 1900s, most people were vigorously active five to ten hours each day. Forty percent of all people lived on farms then, and 80% of all farmwork was done with human labor. Most non-farmworkers did manual work in factories and shops. Even people who did nonphysical work usually walked to their jobs and did heavy chores at home.

This, of course, has changed. Technology has freed most of us from hard labor, but it has imprisoned us within lifestyles that are more conducive to fatness than fitness. This is our reward for progress—and our punishment.

Despite these changes in our lifestyles, though, we are still strongly influenced by powerful urges that have existed since antiquity, exhorting us to eat a pleasurable and satisfying diet.

As a result, eating habits that were once the norm are now considered pathological. People who eat only slightly too much, over a long period of time, now frequently become so overweight that they are labeled as gluttons.

Despite these powerful evolutionary forces, most people try extremely hard to match their caloric intake with their energy needs, and they sacrifice bravely to shed extra pounds. For months and even years at a time, they wage war against their own natural appetites.

However, as time wears on, and physical and psychological hunger makes every passing day more difficult, only about 10% of all people—the strongest of the strong—endure. The rest just can't hold out.

When the holdout is over, most people gain significantly more weight than they had lost, because the "starvation effect" caused by low-calorie dieting triggers caloric hoarding, causing an apple to become almost as fattening as a piece of apple pie once was. In addition, denial-based diets wreak havoc upon the hormones that control hunger and satiety, such as grhelin and leptin, making hunger more intense and more frequent than ever before.

Causing hunger, though, isn't the only major shortcoming of even the best of the conventional denial-based diets.

Denial diets—which means virtually *all* existing weight loss diets—also have these destructive liabilities:

Low-calorie diets often forsake necessary nutrients, most notably protein. When not enough dietary protein is available, the body begins to digest its own protein-packed muscles for energy and nutrients. Micronutrients are also commonly neglected, including those that help break down fat (such as the omega-3 oils), and those that help stabilize blood sugar and control hunger (such as chromium). These nutritional shortfalls debilitate the body and cause food cravings.

Low-carbohydrate diets often compensate for carbohydrate avoidance with excess intake of high-triglyceride fats and dietary proteins, which can harm the cardiovascular system, kidneys, liver, gallbladder, and other organs. High-fat foods, of course, can also be fattening.

Low-fat diets are usually too high in carbohydrates. This causes excessive insulin production, which signals the body to store more energy as body fat. This extra insulin production also overworks the organs that manufacture insulin and can trigger the conditions that lead to diabetes.

Diets that rely on stimulants and appetite suppressants can cause serious damage. At least a hundred people have died recently from using the common herbal diet stimulant ephedra, and many other people have died from taking pharmaceutical diet pills. These diets are also notoriously ineffective for long-term weight management.

Most existing diets are complicated, requiring careful measuring of calories and nutrient grams, purchase of special foods, and restriction of many restaurant foods.

In place of these stringent, unbalanced diets, what's long been needed is a rich, varied, satisfying nutritional program, dense in nutrients—but somehow moderate in calories. Sounds impossible, I know.

But, finally, it's not.

Even so, you may be thinking: "So *what* if weight control is tough? What's the real harm to people? Just not looking good in jeans?"

Here's the harm: Obesity kills. Eating too much accounts for approximately 300,000 deaths per year—about seven times as many as auto accidents. It is the second leading killer in modern American life, after smoking, and will be the leading killer by 2010, if current rates continue.

The process of obesity-related death isn't pretty. Often, before people die, they suffer the amputations of limbs due to weight-related diabetes, or they become blind from that disease. Many others are left crippled from heart disease that was caused by overeating, or develop malignancies linked to dietary excess.

There's a terrible emotional toll, too. The lives of far too many people are devalued by others just because they're overweight. These people are mocked, humiliated, discriminated against, ignored, and held in contempt. Many are denied love. This is not out of the ordinary. It is common.

Perhaps it has happened to you.

A NEW MEDICAL STRATEGY

It had happened to my first patient of the day.

Peggy was a lovely young woman, but over the past few years, after she'd become sedentary due to an auto injury, her weight had surged an extra 60 pounds, and was not easily accommodated on her five-foot-two frame. For the first time in her life, Peggy had become ashamed of herself. The way she was dressed—in dark and baggy clothes—seemed to say, "Don't look at me."

And she was scared. Diabetes ran rampant in her family, and my medical workup indicated that Peggy was, even at age 28, becoming vulnerable to its early onset.

"I need to go on a diet," she said softly, her eyes fixed on the floor.

"I don't believe in weight-loss diets anymore."

Peggy sighed, deep and long, and I could almost hear the hope whoosh out of her.

"I have a new approach," I said. "But it's not a diet. It's a medical strategy, based on a new formulation."

"A pill? I won't take diet pills."

"This isn't a diet pill. It's a completely novel approach. It's a diet, but it's even more than that. It's a medical strategy. I think it's a brilliant one."

I told Peggy about starch blockers. Her face began to brighten.

■

Starch blockers are, in my opinion—and in the opinions of a growing number of academicians and clinicians—*the most significant scientific breakthrough thus far in the history of weight management.* Their development and clinical testing—performed primarily at Mayo Clinic, the University of Scranton, Osaka University, and UCLA-affiliated hospitals—has taken almost thirty years, but the formulation has proven to be abundantly worth the wait.

Starch blockers are a natural, nonprescription partial protein, derived from white kidney beans. This organic plant protein has an extremely unique action. It selectively joins with the enzyme alpha amylase, which digests starch. While this starch-digesting enzyme is bound to the starch blocker, it is temporarily unavailable to break down starch. This condition lasts for about an hour. During that time, approximately two-thirds to three-fourths of the starch that is eaten passes through the digestive system in whole-molecule form, without releasing any calories. Throughout the process of caloric assimilation, the starch calories remain undigested, the same way indigestible fiber does.

Because the starch blocker neutralizes only starch, it doesn't stop the digestion and assimilation of all the other nutrients in starchy foods. The vitamins, minerals, enzymes, and proteins in grains and vegetables are all absorbed.

The biochemical action of the starch blockers is rarely noticed by the people who take them. There are no significant side effects. But what a difference this amazing action makes! Most people eat about one-fourth to one-third of their diets as starch, so almost 25% to 33% of all caloric intake can be neutralized. Instantly. And safely.

There has not previously been a weight management strategy so elegantly simple, so dramatically effective, or so safe to employ.

The beauty of this approach is that it recognizes the power of the natural human desire to eat, and does not try to subvert, alter, or deny this urge. Therefore, this is the first *realistic* weight management program—the only one that deals with people the way they are, instead of the way they should be. It's the first one that relies upon the power of science rather than upon the willpower of people.

Of course, in the best of all worlds, people would have enough willpower to be forever healthy, wealthy, and wise. But that's not how the real world works, is it? And since it's not, should people have to suffer? I don't think so. Not when science can help.

It's very possible, I told Peggy, that future generations will look back on this advance in weight control science with the same respect with which we now regard antibiotics and vaccinations. Those breakthroughs helped end the contagious disease epidemics of the last century, just as starch blockers may help end the degenerative disease epidemics of this century.

The starch blocker diet goes beyond dieting. Diet is the central part of it, but it's a three-step process, consisting of: (1) **redistributing calories to the starchy foods component of the diet; (2) taking emotional control over food; and (3) exercising.**

Thus, the starch blocker diet is really a comprehensive, three-step program.

Furthermore, when you use starch blockers as the central element of this program, they have powerful effects upon *each* of the program's three steps.

- They dramatically reduce the calories that have been redistributed to the starchy foods segment of the diet.
- They heighten emotional control over food by obliterating food cravings and helping stabilize mood chemistry.
- They supercharge exercise by significantly increasing the body's ability to burn fat through physical activity.

Thus, due to the absolutely unique actions of the starch blocker, this approach is even more than a comprehensive program. **It is, in fact, a medical strategy: the starch blocker strategy.**

There's nothing else like it in the field of bariatric medicine.

BREAKING THE SPIRAL OF HIGH-CARB WEIGHT GAIN

As I finished my brief introduction, Peggy's eyes were wide. "It sounds too good to be true," she said. "Imagine! Life beyond dieting!"

"It's just good science and good sense," I replied. "There's nothing mystical or magical about it. It's simply a biochemical strategy for burning your body's fat by reducing the calories coming in from starch."

"So I still get to eat pasta and bread?"

I nodded, and she flashed her first smile of the day. Peggy was from a large Italian family that got together often, and their feasts of spaghetti, ravioli, manicotti, and garlic bread were a central part of their socializing. From my study of psychology, I've learned to appreciate the importance of food in family rituals. For some people, who center their family lives around mealtimes, food *is* family.

But emotion was not the only force driving Peggy's desire for high-carb foods. She was also, in a very real sense, *physically addicted* to carbohydrates. She was caught in America's most common current cause of obesity: the *spiral of carb-related weight gain.*

As recently as ten years ago, starchy carbohydrates, and particularly grains, were still considered by many people in academia and in the diet industry to be the perfect food for weight loss. Grain is low in sugar, free of fat and cholesterol, and can be high in fiber. Tens of millions of people have followed the federal Food Pyramid guidelines that call for extremely high consumption of grains—up to 40% of daily caloric intake. Countless people are still on this starch binge.

But it's been a public health disaster! Most people just aren't biologically equipped to thrive on grain-based diets. The main reason for this is that grains have been widely eaten by humans for only the last *one percent* of human evolutionary history. This relatively short period just hasn't given evolution enough time to reengineer the human body to thrive on starch.

Like it or not, we're stuck with the human anatomy we now have, simply because evolution is so excruciatingly slow. Consider the fact that humans still have tailbones.

The human body, as it's now constructed, runs poorly on starch for a simple reason: *Starch burns too quickly.* It often burns just as fast as sugar and is notoriously disruptive to the metabolism when it's eaten in large amounts.

The body does best with just a moderate amount of starch—about 10% to 15% of caloric intake. We simply can't afford to keep tossing down starch calories the way we have been, or the obesity epidemic will never end.

Our overconsumption has created America's worst current nutritional problem: the four-stage spiral of carb-related weight gain. This spiral starts with the common inability to thrive on carbohydrates—and ends with diabetes.

Here is how the spiral unfolds—and how the starch blocker strategy can stop it.

Stage #1: Hypoglycemia

Carbohydrates—which can be either starch or sugar—are one of the three basic categories of foods, along with protein and fat. Unlike protein and fat, though, which contain components the body uses to rebuild itself (such as amino acids and fatty acids), carbs have only one function. They serve as fuel. That's it. Starch and sugar provide nothing else.

They are the body's first-line source of fuel because they are so chemically similar to blood sugar, or glucose. It takes almost no effort for the body to produce glucose from various sugars, such as sucrose (table sugar) or lactose (milk sugar). These sugars sprint right into your system. Surprisingly, though, the calories from refined starch often hit the system as quickly as those from pure sugar, because the body turns starch into sugar almost immediately. Some of it turns to sugar while it's still in the mouth!

These carb calories smash into the system like a flash flood, triggering a trio of reactions that initially feels good. (1) Blood sugar rockets. (2) Endorphins—the body's own, natural opiates—spike upward. (3) Serotonin, the contentment neurotransmitter, booms. These three actions create the famous "sugar rush," which really should be called a "carb rush," since refined starch is just as potent as sugar.

Sadly, people pay an exorbitant price for this ephemeral high: a long-lasting rebound low that makes them feel weak, hungry, and irritable.

Most people suffer this distress frequently. Anytime they eat too many carbs—which happens often, in our society—they soon suffer an energy slump, and often overeat to compensate for it. This is a problem for *most* of us, because almost all of us are attracted to the rich, satisfying taste of high-carb foods, and the quick energy they provide.

For a huge segment of the population—about 40% of all people—this problem is devastating. It occurs so often, and with so much intensity, that these people are considered to be "carbohydrate intolerant." For them, carbs are almost like a drug—one they just can't handle. They inherit this condition, or develop it by overindulging in carbs.

When people who are carbohydrate intolerant eat too many carbs, it causes wild fluctuations in their levels of the hormone insulin, which moves blood sugar out of the bloodstream and into the cells, where it provides energy. A meal that's heavy in carbs can cause insulin to increase tenfold in just minutes. These insulin swings are a disaster, because they cause energy and mood swings.

When insulin is stable, blood sugar flows into cells at a steady rate, and people tend to feel good: energetic, upbeat, and *not* hungry.

When people eat too many carbs, though, they jump on a roller coaster of highs and lows—*especially* if they're carbohydrate intolerant. One minute they feel fine. Then suddenly they start to feel weak, anxious, and hungry. Time for lunch! A snack! Anything!

The first stage of this insulin instability is known as hypoglycemia, or low blood sugar. That's what Peggy had. Anytime she ate too many carbohydrates—which was practically every day—she went into a frenzy of insulin production, producing even more of it than most people would. This flood of insulin rushed all of her blood sugar into her cells, making her feel great—for a few minutes. Then—*bang!*—her depleted blood sugar, sapped of its energy source, would be incapable of providing her cells with any more power.

When this point hit—as it did for Peggy practically every afternoon around three—it destroyed her willpower. "It slams me into the ground," was the way she put it.

When she felt "slammed down," she invariably ate more carbs—usually a whole wheat bagel. It seemed like an innocent snack, and it helped her feel better. Unfortunately, the boost didn't even last until dinner. By five-thirty, she was usually munching breadsticks, or sampling her dinner as she prepared it.

I could tell Peggy had a carb problem just by looking at her. She had what's called trunkal obesity, characterized by a puffy abdomen. This type of "apple shape" obesity is far more common among people with carbohydrate intolerance and insulin problems than is "pear shape" obesity (or peripheral obesity), which is characterized by heavy thighs and hips.

As with most people with trunkal obesity, the fat in Peggy's stomach area usually came on quickly. She said she could literally feel her abdominal fat, including her "love handles," bloat up right after a starchy meal.

But the good news for Peggy—and maybe for you, too—is that this carbohydrate-caused fat can leave the abdomen almost as quickly as it comes, if the starch blocker strategy is employed. Easy on—easy off.

Nobody's sure why carbohydrate weight sticks first to the stomach area, or why it comes and goes so quickly. The best theory, though, is that evolution dictated that people needed a quick-burning source of stored fat for short-term hunger problems.

The starch blocker strategy is perfect for helping end obesity due to carbohydrate and insulin problems. By flattening the curve of carb-calorie consumption, it can stop the four-stage spiral of high-carb weight gain before it ever gets started.

I knew that the starch blocker strategy would probably make Peggy's life almost instantly better. It would stabilize her energy, improve her mood, stop her food cravings, and control her hunger. Even more important, though, it would probably prevent terrible problems later on.

Hypoglycemia is often just the very beginning of people's problems with carbohydrates. Left unchecked, hypoglycemia gradually progresses to the next stage in the spiral of carb-related weight gain: hyperglycemia, or *high* blood sugar.

Stage #2: Hyperglycemia

Hyperglycemia is horrible. Having it is almost like having permanent hypoglycemia.

Hyperglycemia starts after people chronically overeat carbs and overproduce insulin for a long period of time. This chronic overproduction not only depletes their supplies of insulin, but it also causes their cells to become resistant to the actions of insulin. The cells develop tolerance to insulin, in somewhat the same way that the cells of heroin addicts develop tolerance to opiates, requiring ever higher amounts.

Hyperglycemia eventually strikes up to an estimated 25% of all people, generally as they approach midlife, and is a crucial factor in our epidemic of overweight.

When hyperglycemia occurs, too much blood sugar just sits sluggishly in the bloodstream as cells literally begin to starve. These cells send out distress signals, interpreted by the brain as hunger and irritation. As a rule, people try to get rid of these feelings by eating, but that only solves the problem partially and temporarily. Other common quick fixes for this situation are caffeine (because it boosts insulin) and nicotine (because it restores calmness).

Even with these temporary corrections, though, the body and brain are still temporarily deprived of adequate blood sugar, causing widespread damage and death to cells. In fact, becoming hungry and weak from hyperglycemia—*or from a low-calorie diet,* which also starves the brain—kills almost as many brain cells as getting drunk. That's one of the dirty little secrets of the diet industry.

People often put up with hyperglycemia for years at a time—gaining weight despite their best efforts—buoyed only by the belief that things can't get much worse. But they can.

Syndrome X can strike.

Stage #3: Syndrome X

Syndrome X is a recently discovered condition that hits when hyperglycemia combines with carbohydrate intolerance, insulin resistance, high levels of blood fats, and excess body fat. This dangerous combination of factors comes together in approximately 20% of all middle-aged people and makes weight loss almost impossible for them. Any one of these five factors is terribly disruptive to normal metabolism, but when they gang together, they overwhelm the body. They keep blood sugar out of the cells—including the brain cells—

to a dangerous degree. The only way to temporarily relieve Syndrome X symptoms is to overeat, and literally *force* blood sugar into cells, but this just makes the problem worse in the long run.

Not recognized until 1988, Syndrome X is now considered one of the largest epidemics ever to befall America, according to a recent article in the *Journal of the American Medical Association (JAMA)*. It's a classic result of affluence, uncommon in poor countries, and believed to be relatively rare in America until recent decades.

Like the conditions that lead to it, Syndrome X is badly exacerbated by eating too many carbohydrates—which is, unfortunately, exactly what millions of people do in order to fight the noxious symptoms of the problem. It's like throwing fuel on a fire.

Even when the various factors composing Syndrome X do not become severe, they can still combine to become a major cause of weight gain. A great many midlife people suffer at least mild, subclinical Syndrome X, often without knowing it. They usually say, "Oh, my metabolism must be slowing down." But weight gain from metabolic slowing is mostly myth. The metabolism only slows by about 1% per decade, and that's not enough to account for notable weight gain. The real culprit in midlife weight gain is the constellation of factors that comprise Syndrome X.

This condition kills cells throughout the body and brain and is a major precursor of many degenerative diseases, including cardiovascular disease, cancer, and Alzheimer's.

It is most closely linked, though, to the final step in the degenerative spiral of carb-related weight gain: diabetes.

Stage #4: Diabetes

About 10% of the U.S. population has diabetes, and more than one-third of them don't even realize it. These undiagnosed people know they don't feel good, but their symptoms are so similar to those of Syndrome X—and even to mild Syndrome X—that they just take them for granted. They know they're hungry much of the time, and that they often get weak and irritable before meals, but they think, "That's life—almost everybody feels this way."

Everybody doesn't. Not even all diabetics feel like this. Some of them control the disease carefully, limiting their intake of carbohydrates to a spartan degree. When they do, it helps reduce symptoms of the disease.

Obviously, though, this degree of denial can be a terrible burden. It's so difficult that millions of people just can't do it, and suffer horrendous consequences. Blindness. Amputations. Kidney failure. Nerve disease. Death.

Diabetes, in our current carb-obsessed era, is more common than ever, and it is striking ever younger people—even children. In fact, diabetes is now so prevalent among kids that the name of the obesity-related type of the disease has been changed from Adult Onset diabetes to Type II diabetes.

Starch blockers offer great promise even to people with diabetes. This was demonstrated in studies at Mayo Clinic and in Japan. These studies indicated that starch blockers may be able to allow people with diabetes to enjoy much more normal eating patterns—while actually *reducing* the degree of their complications from diabetes.

The implications of this are astonishing. It probably represents the most important advance against diabetes since the introduction of insulin treatment. Perhaps even *more* momentous is the realistic possibility that starch blockers may help *prevent* the onset of diabetes.

If widespread prevention of America's fifth-ranked killer occurs—and we firmly believe it can—this organic substance will become entrenched as one of natural medicine's most important new protocols.

■

As you probably know, a legion of insulin-stabilizing, weight control programs has already been created to try to stop this four-stage progression. Each has been announced with great fanfare, each touting a twist: reliance on protein, reliance on fat, on strenuous exercise, on pharmaceutical drugs, on appetite suppressants—even reliance on religion.

But each has failed for the majority of people trying it.

None has realistically dealt with people the way they really are:

flawed in biochemistry, with greater personal agendas than centering their lives on dieting.

Thus, the starch blocker strategy represents an entirely new paradigm in weight management.

■

"This all sounds so . . . different," Peggy said.

That was an understatement. This weight control strategy is absolutely unique, different from all of the diets that have ever been created.

FIVE BIG DIFFERENCES

Here are the major differences in the starch blocker strategy, in order of importance.

1. **This is the first nondenial weight program.**

   - You can eat a normal amount of food, *without* assimilating all the calories.
   - Eliminating starch calories allows consumption of relatively more calories from proteins, fats, and sugars.
   - You can eat satisfying gourmet dishes on this program— such as those provided in this book by famous French chef Philippe Boulot—rather than low-calorie, low-carb diet foods that often taste like "rabbit food."

2. **This is the first no-hunger weight program.**

   - Abdominal fullness, caused by calorie-neutralized starchy foods, activates the "stretch receptors" in the stomach that help turn off physical hunger.
   - Insulin stability, achieved by blocking starch calories, stops blood sugar and insulin swings, and the hunger that they cause.
   - Being able to freely enjoy delicious starchy foods—and to add some nonstarch calories—eliminates psychological hunger.

3. **This is the first weight program that safely directs the body to burn stored fat.**

   - Unlike *low-calorie* diets, this new strategy doesn't break down muscle tissue by restricting protein, and it doesn't starve the body of other necessary nutrients.
   - Unlike *low-carbohydrate* diets, it doesn't call for abundant consumption of high-fat foods, which can hurt health.
   - Unlike *low-fat* diets, it doesn't call for high intake of carbohydrates, which can disrupt insulin stability.
   - This approach makes exercise burn body fat more efficiently. It supercharges exercise by reducing stored carbohydrates, which the body must deplete before it can burn body fat.

4. **This is the first weight management approach that appears capable of relieving complications from diabetes.**

   - This strategy can help to arrest some of the symptoms of diabetes.
   - This strategy has been shown to control the precursor conditions of diabetes, including hypoglycemia, hyperglycemia, and Syndrome X.

5. **This is the first weight program that has neither physical nor psychological side effects.**

   - It doesn't employ general stimulants, metabolic stimulants, or appetite suppressants.
   - It doesn't raise cholesterol or other blood fats, as do some *low-carb,* high-fat diets.
   - It doesn't destabilize insulin levels, as do some *low-fat,* high-carb diets.
   - It has been certified 100% free of physical side effects by researchers employed by the National Institutes of Health.
   - It doesn't contribute to a psychological sense of deprivation.
   - It can actually improve mood chemistry by stopping the blood sugar and hormonal fluctuations that cause mood swings.

Peggy had tried all the diets that didn't offer these five big differences, and she felt she'd failed. She hadn't. The diets had.

For Peggy, though, the long years of failure were about to end. In the next chapter, I'll tell you about her success, and about the successes of the other two patients I saw on this special day.

A major reason that they all succeeded, I believe, was because I didn't demand denial.

Denial diets, which are the heart and soul of the diet industry, are no more suited to real human behavior than is trying to get through the day by breathing as little air as possible, or drinking as little water as possible. They sap the pleasure from life, disrupt the metabolism, and demand that people become full-time dieters, forever focused on abstinence.

This does not mean, of course, that the starch blocker strategy is one long Mardi Gras of indulgence. It requires effort, patience, and self-control.

However, it offers inestimable advantages over denial diets. It makes adjustments for the biochemical vulnerabilities of the human metabolism, and it allows for the existence of normal psychological drives. It sparks a fire of empowerment that ignites the human will. It works *for* people—the way they really are—instead of against their natural urges.

I have already seen this happen, in just my own patients, many, many times.

And this is just the beginning—the very beginning—of the new era of weight management.

TWO

THE DISCOVERY

Changing the Field of Weight Management Forever

need some diet pills!" my second patient of the day said, the moment he sat down.

Norm was frustrated. At 45, he was about 35 pounds overweight, despite the fact that he ate moderately and exercised strenuously for an hour every day.

That should have been enough, right? But it wasn't.

An hour a day of rigorous exercise is more than most people do, but you've got to remember that even your very recent ancestors did four, five, or maybe even ten times that much. We live in a new world of declining physical activity—but our caloric intake has hardly declined at all. In fact, many people are eating far more calories than their ancestors ever did, because they're more affluent, and because of the advent of fast food and highly processed food.

Fast food was Norm's downfall, even though his only restaurant meal of the day was lunch. That one meal of junk food, though, added about 300 unnecessary calories to his daily total. Every ten days, those extra calories added up to about a pound of body fat— some of which Norm worked off, and some of which he didn't.

I refused to give Norm the diet pills he wanted. I told him that they just don't work over the long run, and they have too many side effects. I never gave in to the Fen-Phen fad, and after people started dying from it, and developing serious heart and lung problems from even minimal use, I was glad I'd been so adamant.

I also told Norm he would have to cut out his burger and fries for lunch, because his cholesterol was too high, and because he was already hyperglycemic. The extra fats and starches were pushing him ever closer to Syndrome X, the last stop before diabetes.

A year earlier, another doctor had put Norm on a low-fat, anticholesterol diet, but he'd abandoned it because, as restrictive as it was, it hadn't helped his weight. That's very common. People rarely lose weight on low-cholesterol diets, because they usually just end up substituting high-carb foods for high-fat foods. Their cholesterol often drops, but their weight—which is an even bigger general risk factor than cholesterol—typically stays the same, or even goes up.

By the time I broached the subject of burgers, Norm wasn't very happy with me. Like so many patients, he was tired of doctors who made difficult demands without offering much assistance. But then I told him about the diet that he'd be able to eat on the starch blocker strategy, and his attitude changed. For once, he was going to get some real help.

I recommended that he take two starch blockers with every meal. Because each starch blocker neutralizes about 400 starch calories, that would be sufficient to block most of the starch he ate. The supplements would cost him about a dollar a day.

Norm left with new hope. His long hours of exercise, he believed, were finally going to pay off.

■

My last patient of the day, Gina, was in the midst of one of the worst times for weight gain among women—her early sixties, just past menopause, when her estrogen was no longer helping her burn stored fat. Prior to menopause, when estrogen is abundant, women tend to burn fat more easily, presumably because this assists in child-rearing functions, such as breast-feeding.

Because Gina's 30 extra pounds of fat were hormonally related, most of it was stored in her hips and thighs, where it would be more resistant to loss than fat stored in the abdomen. But even this type of peripheral, pear-shaped obesity responds to starch blockers. It just takes longer.

Not inordinately longer, though. I expected Gina to lose about one and one-half pounds per week, compared to about two pounds per week for Peggy and Norm. Of course, all three of them could have lost weight much faster with more aggressive employment of the starch blocker strategy, but I didn't want them to. Losing more than two pounds per week triggers the starvation effect of caloric hoarding and destabilizes the hormones of hunger and satiety, making rebound weight gain far more likely. Fast weight loss, I told Gina, is a sucker's game.

She was disappointed. Common reaction. Lots of patients want to lose weight quickly. But once they start the starch blocker strategy, their disappointment fades. As soon as they discover how comfortable the strategy is, they realize that there's generally only one good reason for wanting to lose weight fast: *Diets don't feel good.* The sooner they're over, the better.

Of course, diet promoters also know that denial diets are painful, so they feed into this fixation on FAST FAST FAST!—as if people are just too *impatient* to wait for weight loss.

But—think about it—people really aren't all that impatient. They wait for Christmas, for their vacations, for retirement, for the weekend, for raises—for any number of things. They're just impatient with things that *hurt*. Such as hunger.

Gina's patience, I thought, would be bolstered by the fact that she would feel better almost immediately. She was in the difficult early days of Syndrome X, and was almost certain to feel a huge boost in well-being after her insulin levels stabilized. For most people, starch blockers are great for stopping mood swings.

I loaded Gina down with information packets and handouts. Much of it was material that you'll now find in this book: how starch blockers work; results of studies; the history of starch blockers; the best ways to use them; what they will do and won't do; how to use them as part of an integrated program of diet, psychological empowerment, and exercise; how to determine starch contents of various foods; how to prepare tasty calorie-neutralized recipes; and more.

Gina was somewhat overwhelmed by all the information. Even so, she was relieved. She'd come in thinking that I was going to put her on a denial diet and make her life harder. But I was making it easier.

That made me feel great. To be honest, I felt great not just for Gina—and for Peggy and Norm—but for me, too.

For years, I'd struggled to find a way to solve this common, deadly problem. My struggle had taken me on a journey—geographic as well as intellectual—that had been exhausting and often baffling. Now that journey was over.

As my day wound down, I strolled through my clinic, which is quite different from that of most doctors. My treatment center, in the breezy, ocean-cooled environs of Los Angeles' UCLA area, has offices for a wide range of integrative health specialists: acupuncturists, nutritionists, chiropractors, exercise physiologists, and counselors. We even have a large exercise room filled with fitness equipment that we use to demonstrate various workout programs.

The clinic—with its emphasis on integrative treatment—is a reflection of my journey. And on this day, which would once have frustrated me to the point of despair, what I saw around me—caring professionals using cutting-edge protocols—made me feel very good. The journey had been worth it.

MY JOURNEY

I've always been attracted to seemingly insoluble problems. Maybe I'm just a masochist. But I really think I'm more of an optimist, somebody who thinks that sooner or later almost *any* problem can be solved. That's why I was initially drawn to weight management. Like other enigmatic problems I've become fascinated with—most notably autism and chronic pain—I just couldn't believe there wasn't a solution to it somewhere.

If I had known that it would take more than thirty years to find that solution, though, I'm not sure I would have ever gotten started. Thank God for ignorance—it gets us going on problems we'd otherwise be afraid to tackle.

My first pass at the problem, though, was a miserable failure. In the late 1960s, I was a young M.A. in psychology, and like many people who have recently begun to specialize, I saw the world through the lens of my own specialty. Many physical problems, I felt, had powerful psychological roots. Surely, weight control was one. Overeating was an emotional problem, wasn't it? A stress reaction? An attempt to stuff down feelings with food?

Nice theories—but they went nowhere. You could counsel people until you were blue in the face, and they'd still be fat.

I experienced the same lack of success—using just psychology—with other problems I'd become interested in during grad school, such as autism. At that time, many people still thought autism was primarily an emotional disorder. That didn't seem to apply, though, to the autistic children with whom I was working. Something was wrong physiologically—I just knew it.

Therefore, as I continued to work toward my doctorate in psychology, I gravitated to the new field of physiological psychology—the exploration of the nexus of mind and body. The mind/body approach was in its infancy back then, and seemed to offer solutions to a wide range of problems, including weight management.

Even so, nothing I learned seemed to help people with serious weight problems. Many of them were able to lose weight temporarily with the help of strict diets and concurrent counseling, but it was often torture for them, practically a full-time job.

I wasn't having much luck with autism, either. The truth is, neither I nor others have yet made significant strides with that disorder. However, I did come across a tantalizing lead that took me down a strange new path. I noticed that autistic children seemed impervious to pain, so I started studying pain management, and the brand-new theory of endorphin output.

This prompted me to follow up on rumors about an arcane form of pain control used by a few members of L.A.'s Asian community. I had never previously heard of this method. Virtually no one in America had. It was called acupuncture.

As I researched this mysterious and sometimes miraculous method, I met a man who changed my life forever. Ju Gim Shek was a doctor of Oriental Medicine—the first I'd ever met. He told me that there was a milieu of medicine—of which acupuncture was a part—that was neither physiological nor psychological, but instead revolved around esoteric energy fields. He preached a protocol of energy balance that was foreign to everything I'd ever learned. It certainly seemed to work, though, and appealed to the pragmatist in me.

Even the way he administered his practice was different. He treated sick patients for free—and billed people only when they were healthy. "The true aim of a doctor," he told me, "is to treat *before* illness."

Fascinated, I traveled to Asia and gained admission to the prestigious Hong Kong College of Acupuncture. After years of study, I became an Oriental Medicine doctor, or O.M.D., and was the first Westerner ever licensed to practice acupuncture in America. I founded the UCLA School of Medicine's acupuncture program and later became a commissioner of accreditation for all U.S. acupuncture and Oriental Medicine programs. Since that time, acupuncture has been widely accepted by American pain specialists as a first-line treatment for chronic and acute pain.

For some time, I thought acupuncture would also unlock the mysteries of weight control, because of its influence upon the autonomic nervous system. Over time, my optimism dwindled. Acupuncture helped, yes—just not enough. Only people who were highly motivated responded with permanent weight loss.

I also prescribed potent Chinese herbal medicines to some of my weight management patients. Same lack of dramatic results. The only people who did well were those who put great effort into it. That wasn't good enough. Patients shouldn't have to do all the work. *Science* should do some of the heavy lifting.

As the 1970s progressed and Western medicine began increasingly to integrate natural modalities into its treatments, I was drawn to medical school. I was impressed by the aggressive approach of Western medicine, and by its increasingly sophisticated use of technology.

Even after I became an M.D., though, I was still skeptical of conventional medicine's infatuation with pharmaceutical drugs, which are still the mainstay of most doctors' practices. For long-standing lifestyle problems, such as weight control, pharmaceutical drugs just aren't appropriate. Too invasive. Too many side effects. They may work well for a few months, but most people can't tolerate them for a lifetime. Permanent control of lifestyle problems requires natural, noninvasive approaches, which adjust the body's normal functions without commandeering them.

As the 1980s dawned, I first heard about a remarkable new non-pharmaceutical substance for weight control. It was called starch blockers. I initially read about it in a journal edited by the coauthor of this book, health science author Cameron Stauth. Starch blockers appeared to hold great promise. They were natural, but powerful. They worked *with* the body's natural functions, instead of against them.

Starch blockers were briefly introduced to the market—prematurely, I felt—and caused a wave of interest. After several months, though, the few brands that existed were removed from the market by the FDA, because they had a strong, druglike effect, but had not yet gone through the FDA's lengthy drug approval process. More testing was mandated, even though about ten years of research had already gone into their development.

For another fifteen years, new rounds of tests—described in detail in the next chapter—were performed at universities and hospitals in America and abroad, as the product was perfected and as its safety and efficacy were proven. The process was painstaking, but good science is always slow.

During this time, I became active in sports medicine because I was fascinated by the health strategies of world-class athletes. As a member of the 1984 Olympic Games Medical Advisory Commission, I discovered that even many athletes had to fight weight gain—especially those who were trying to subsist on the then relatively new government guidelines that called for high carb consumption.

Hungry for new perspectives, I pursued part of my medical studies at hospitals in England, to study some of the progressive new approaches that were being introduced in Europe. In the United States, we often think that America's medicine is the world's medicine, but that's a naively parochial perspective. Western Europe, in particular, has some of the finest research hospitals in the world, which have an exemplary record of introducing innovative protocols. While I was there, for example, many of the best early AIDS drugs were being developed. Europe is also a hotbed of new integrative approaches.

In England, I broadened my expertise to include classic Western herbology, as well as homeopathy, the naturalistic approach that has been likened to inoculation.

Both these approaches, I found, could help with weight control, but they just didn't have the specificity needed to home in on the heart of the problem. By the 1990s, it had become clear that the primary cause of weight gain in our current culture is carbohydrate overload—because of the metabolic damage it does—and no herb or homeopathic remedy can resolve that.

Even so, a multitude of patients kept coming to me with the same old problem—weight gain—complicated by the endless array of conditions it contributes to: heart disease, stroke, atherosclerosis, arteriosclerosis, diabetes, Syndrome X, certain cancers, cirrhosis of the liver, sleep apnea, back pain, arthritic complications, and psychological stress.

It was easy to tell patients what they *should* do—cut way back on carb calories—but could I do the same if I were them? I've always been naturally thin, so I'll never know.

It was discouraging to see so many people whom I could not help. I often felt as powerless as they did.

Then, one afternoon less than a year ago, I was talking to UCLA-affiliated researcher Jay Udani, M.D., who wrote the introduction to this book, and he mentioned starch blockers. The necessary testing of them had almost been completed, he said, and the results of the existing clinical studies were extremely impressive. The bright promise born in 1980 had been more than fulfilled. Starch blockers now met the current FDA standards, which had been modified somewhat in 1994 to allow the public better access to natural products. Soon, Dr. Udani predicted, almost everyone in America would know about starch blockers.

I still remember that conversation, the way you remember other turning points of your life.

A difficult journey had ended—and a happy one had just begun.

SUCCESS!

Peggy sat across from me in my office, resplendent in a bright new summer dress.

Over the past six months, many things about her had changed. The way she dressed. The way she held her head high and looked me in the eye. The energy she exuded. The shape of her face—so much more striking, now that it wasn't rounded by fat. And, of course, her body.

She had lost 50 pounds, was still losing, and was down to 115.

"I want to lose two more pounds!" she enthused. "I'm gonna be *skinny!*"

"Quit now. Shift to weight maintenance."

She looked at me like I was Dr. Wet Blanket. "When I'm *this close* to my perfect weight?"

For looks, I told her, two more pounds would be fine. But there's a lot more to weight control than looks. Protruding ribs and starved-look cheekbones might look chic on the cover of *Vogue,* I said, but they're not compatible with robust health. People usually need a couple of extra pounds as an energy reserve, for all those days when they have to skip a meal, or burn more calories than they consume.

Without any significant amount of stored fat, I told Peggy, people often end up running on adrenaline, thyroid hormones, and the stress hormone cortisol—a destructive triad that's otherwise known as nervous energy.

You can get by on nervous energy once in a while, but if you run on empty too often, it will soon exhaust all your hormonal reserves, paving the way to premature aging and a host of chronic and degenerative disorders.

So I told Peggy that every time I pass a rack of magazines featuring emaciated models looking like pretty scarecrows, I feel like buying every issue, just to dump them all in the trash.

"You're not a standard diet doctor, are you?" Peggy said.

"I'll take that as a compliment."

Norm and Gina also had appointments that day, for their six-month check-ins. Norm was first, and I couldn't believe the changes in him. He was wearing a tight cotton tee shirt, and he pulled it up proudly to show me his new "washboard" stomach.

"Man, you've got abs of steel now!" I said.

"I've *always* had abs of steel. But now you can *see* them." I laughed. "I'm serious, I could do two hundred toe-touch sit-ups back when I couldn't even *find* my toes."

He'd lost about 30 of the 35 pounds of fat he'd hoped to lose, and had gained five to ten pounds of muscle, from exercising more.

"Running isn't as hard," he said, "when you're not saddled with a 30-pound pack of blubber."

In addition, his exercise was now more effective because he was carrying far fewer stored carbs, which the body must burn first during exercise before it begins oxidizing body fat (more on this in Chapter Six). Every time he exercised now, he saw a decline in his body fat, and it was encouraging.

Besides, he had much more energy, and simply felt a lot more like exercising.

Peggy, and also Gina, had experienced the same renewed interest in exercise. It was far easier for them, now that they were lighter and had more stable levels of energy. They, too, loved the quick results from exercise that they were seeing. Peggy was jogging for the first time since she'd injured her back in a car accident, and Gina was in an aqua-aerobics class.

Sometimes, patients are surprised when I tell them to exercise, because they expect to be thin just from taking starch blockers. That's not realistic. Nothing that lasts a lifetime is ever caused by just one factor, working on its own.

To be effective, the entire starch blocker strategy must be used. Here are some details on its three steps.

THE STARCH BLOCKER STRATEGY

1. **Redistributing Calories—and Neutralizing Them.** This doesn't mean restricting calories. Because of caloric neutralization, it actually means *adding* them. It means moving a larger percentage of your existing caloric intake to the starch category, to take advantage of caloric blockage. Calories from fats, sugars, and proteins may also be increased moderately, but this increase must not exceed the number of calories that are neutralized. Furthermore, sugar calories must be strictly monitored, since sugar—the equally evil twin of starch—can disrupt glucose and insulin stability. Nonetheless, most people eat more *on* the strategy than off it.

2. **Taking Emotional Control.** One of the most amazing things about the strategy is that it helps give people emotional power over food.

By stabilizing levels of blood sugar and insulin, starch blockers typically free people from the food cravings and mood swings that may long have dictated their eating habits. This glycemic stabilization also helps ensure proper production of calming neurotransmitters (such as serotonin) and energizing hormones (including norepinephrine). These neurological factors empower the human will tremendously. In addition, people get a terrific psychological lift from being able to eat normal foods in normal amounts. Net result: emotional control over eating habits.

3. **Burning Body Fat with Exercise.** Theoretically, exercise isn't necessary, because the patients using starch blockers in the controlled studies were advised not to exercise so that researchers could be sure that starch blockers were the only factor causing weight loss. That's good science—but it's not a good way to live the rest of your life. Exercise not only allows consumption of correspondingly more calories, it also helps keep the cardiovascular system, lungs, bones, and joints healthy, and even benefits other parts of the body that we don't commonly associate with exercise, such as the prostate and breasts, which have a lower incidence of cancer among people who exercise. In addition, exercise helps cognitive function, memory, and mood so much that it is now considered an important hedge against Alzheimer's and major depression. Besides, muscles that aren't exercised become flaccid, and look as flabby as fat. For feeling good, nothing beats fitness. For people participating in the strategy, exercise is easier, and it's more efficient at burning fat. The strategy supercharges exercise.

On the strategy, weight can be expected to come off at about one to two pounds per week, until dieters reach their goal weights. After that, the program can be relaxed somewhat, either by neutralizing fewer starch calories or by eating more nonstarch calories.

In the book's next section, we'll give you all the how-to details on the three steps of the strategy. It's a short section. I'm sure you're excited about getting started, and we want that to happen as quickly as you do.

■

Gina was my last appointment of the day, and my most gratifying. She was healthier, stronger, happier—more alive.

When people think about weight loss, they inevitably fixate upon looks, because of our society's preoccupation with appearance. But looking better is among the most trivial benefits of overcoming obesity (which is defined as being 20% over your ideal weight).

If I were a bariatric physician—specializing in weight control and treating only the condition itself—perhaps I would be more caught up in the common obsession with appearance. These days, though, I practice family medicine, and deal each day with the wreckage of lives that is caused by obesity. When people come to me with cardiovascular disease or diabetes, I don't spend a lot of time telling them how great they'll soon look in their swimsuits.

"What's your weight down to?" I asked Gina.

"I really don't know. I think I reached my goal weight, but my real goal is just to feel better."

"Good for you!" I love that attitude. "How are you doing?"

"Better all the time. My Syndrome X symptoms are practically nonexistent now. I don't get jittery before meals, and I have more energy than I had in my thirties."

Gina left without asking how much longer she needed to stay on the strategy. She already knew. The starch blocker strategy would probably be a part of her life forever—like taking a baby aspirin every day to prevent heart disease, taking glucosamine to control arthritis, or taking antioxidants to slow down aging.

After Gina left, I had a few minutes to myself, with no more patients to see. My caseload is actually a little lighter these days, because a number of my patients are solving their own problems with the starch blocker strategy, often preventing them before they require treatment.

Finally, I have fulfilled the exhortation of my mentor Ju Gim Shek, who long ago counseled me to treat *before* illness.

Occasionally now, at the end of a long and satisfying day—particularly a day that would once have ended in frustration—I'll ask myself, "Is this what that long and difficult journey was all about? This simple solution? This triumph of science?"

THREE

THE SCIENCE

Clinical Proof of Effectiveness

How good is the science behind this?" my patient asked. She was a scientist herself, a cell biologist, and was proud—and rightly so—of her skepticism about new medical trends.

"The science is excellent. Some of it's been done right around here, at UCLA."

"Good. There's *so* much pseudoscience these days."

"I can't argue with that."

Pseudoscience, I have to admit, has long been the bane of my own field, integrative medicine. Far too many alternative protocols have been driven by commercial considerations rather than science. I find this repugnant for a couple of reasons. One: I'm a skeptic myself. Back in the late 1960s, even after I'd seen how powerful acupuncture could be, I didn't fully accept it until I had completed a study on the electrophysical correlates of acupuncture points, research that's still often referred to today. The second reason I hate the shaky science that permeates parts of integrative medicine is quite simple: In my profession, when someone makes a mistake, people can die.

Questionable science is especially rampant in the weight management industry. In 2002, the Federal Trade Commission charged that about half of 300 diet advertisements that were reviewed made at least one false statement. Even after that investigation, though, many of the claims that still continue to be made for weight loss diets and products are ludicrous, such as one that now promises a steady weight loss of ten pounds per week, without cutting calories or exercising.

However, the introduction to the public of starch blockers as a weight management aid has been characterized by a tone that has been quite the opposite of the hyperbole that typically surrounds new weight loss products. One of the primary reasons for this is that for many years during the development of starch blockers, they were not perceived as a weight loss product. Most of the early research on them was aimed at developing a product that could help control diabetes.

That goal still seems within reach. More than ever before, it appears likely that starch blockers will soon prove to be valuable in helping control Type II, non-insulin-dependent diabetes. New clinical trials on this are being undertaken at a UCLA–affiliated hospital and at other institutions.

Because starch blockers offer so much hope for diabetics, they were developed and refined in university laboratories and at major research hospitals, such as Mayo Clinic. In contrast, many other current weight control formulations, which have only the single application of being diet aids, have been developed primarily in marketing department conference rooms. In these situations, an existing substance—such as the stimulating herb ephedra—has often been shoehorned into service as a diet aid despite its scientific inappropriateness. This is an inexpensive way to bring products to the market, but it does not serve science, and it does not serve the public. In the particular case of ephedra, this approach has done great disservice, resulting in deaths and in increased cynicism among the public about weight loss products.

People deserve better. They deserve to hear more than "ten pounds a week without dieting."

They deserve—*you* deserve—to hear about the science that supports the safety and efficacy of the products you put into your body.

Here is a bird's-eye view of the science behind starch blockers.

THE HOWARD HUGHES CONNECTION

Starch blockers were first developed under the direction of the legendary Howard Hughes. In his declining years, the billionaire was best known for his eccentricities, including reclusiveness and an extreme phobia of germs. Before that, though, he was widely recognized as an extraordinary engineering innovator, a keen observer of new sciences, and an ardent supporter of medical research. His group of Howard Hughes Medical Institutes is still one of the finest consortiums of research hospitals in the world.

In 1971, Howard Hughes, or one of his top aides, spotted an article in an obscure scientific journal that would eventually change the direction of weight management. The article described a mystery.

For reasons unknown, mice in an experiment that had been conducted in Venezuela had died of starvation, even though they'd been fed a seemingly nutritious diet. The article said that perhaps some form of "antinutrient" had caused the baffling starvation.

Hughes assigned a team of researchers at Miami's Howard Hughes Medical Institute to look into the mystery. The group was headed by George Thorn, the hospital's director of medical research.

Over the next two years Thorn's research team linked the Venezuelan mystery to existing knowledge about certain antinutrient proteins that inhibit food digestion by binding with the digestive enzymes of insects, animals, and human beings.

It has been known since the 1940s, for example, that raw, unprocessed wheat contains small amounts of a protein that binds with the receptor sites on alpha amylase, the enzyme that digests starch. This makes the amylase temporarily incapable of breaking down starch. The protein stays in the system—"stuck" to the enzyme—for only about an hour. It's quickly moved through the digestive tract, along with the enzyme and the other food substances that were eaten, and is excreted.

While it is in the system, though, it renders amylase incapable of breaking down all of the starch that's present. This undigested starch then passes through the system in whole-molecule form, with the other foodstuffs.

Because the undigested starch stays in whole-molecule form, it does not release any calories. In effect, it becomes much like indigestible fiber, such as that found in bran, lettuce, and other fibrous foods. All indigestible fibers pass through the system without releasing calories.

This enzyme-inhibiting protein helps protect wheat in the field and in storage bins. When insects and animals, such as weevils and mice, scavenge raw wheat, they ingest this protein, which prohibits digestion of some of the starch from the wheat. This discourages insects and animals from eating raw wheat. When they try to live on it, they don't get enough calories, so they tend to abandon it.

Thus, enzyme inhibitors are protective mechanisms born of evolution that enable plants to survive, much the same way that the spines on a cactus or the thorns on a blackberry vine help those plants to survive.

What researchers discovered at the Howard Hughes Medical Institute—and in related research at the University of Miami—was that the plants with the most abundant amounts of this enzyme-inhibiting antinutrient were white kidney beans.

And white kidney beans had primarily composed the diet of the Venezuelan mice that had starved to death. End of mystery.

The researchers named the enzyme-inhibiting substance in white kidney beans "phaseolamin." The word is derived from the Latin word for kidney beans, *phaseo vulgaris,* combined with *am* (short for "amylase") and *in* (short for "inhibitor").

Even today, some medical experts incorrectly assume that phaseolamin is a compound, but it's just a vegetable glycoprotein with a very specific molecular weight. In effect, it's a part of a part of a part of a specific plant protein.

The initial interest in phaseolamin among almost all researchers was as a tool to fight diabetes. Researchers were well aware that eating excessive amounts of starch can be critically injurious to people with diabetes, because it rushes glucose into the bloodstream. They hoped phaseolamin would help curtail this rush.

For several years, during the latter 1970s, they worked on isolating phaseolamin from other substances in kidney beans, especially "lectins," which can cause blood cells to clump together. The researchers were, in a sense, trying to find a standardized, replicable way to pull the "needle" of phaseolamin out of the "haystack" of white kidney beans.

This refinement process was exceptionally difficult. It was easy to just grind up beans, but that left in too many impurities. Ground-up beans did seem to have a moderate enzyme-inhibiting action, but they caused too many side effects, such as bloating and diarrhea.

Unfortunately, this did not stop some of the people who had been researching starch blockers from rushing them to market. In

1982, crude bean extracts began to appear on the market and were sold for weight loss. Sales of these products were strong, and for several months these crude "starch blockers" became a new fad.

A couple of reputable laboratories joined the effort, and did manage to produce pure starch blockers that were generally effective, although expensive. However, the market was dominated by the cheaper, impure, ineffective products; which were markedly inferior to today's vastly improved version of the product.

The Food and Drug Administration quickly intervened. They ruled that it wasn't legal for retailers to claim that all of these "starch blockers" caused weight loss. To do so would be a health claim, and at that time, the only products that could make health claims were drugs.

When retailers could no longer sell starch blockers explicitly for weight control, almost all American companies lost interest in the approach. For them, it was like trying to sell Diet Pepsi without being able to mention that it was calorie-free. However, two companies that had adequate refining processes did continue to market them, without any promotion, and they remained moderately popular in a few other countries, including Italy.

In 1983, the *Journal of the American Medical Association* published a study in which researchers tested the effectiveness of several of the most popular, old, crude bean extract products that had been sold for weight loss. Predictably, they exerted only a minimal degree of enzyme inhibition, which resulted in negligible weight loss. The article concluded, quite accurately, that these crude bean extracts were not efficacious. When that article appeared, most of the research community lost interest in starch blockers.

Not Mayo Clinic, though. Doctors there, led by Eugene P. DiMagno, M.D., continued to investigate the potential of starch blockers for helping diabetics. Unlike most other researchers at that time, they did not accept at face value the conclusion of the *JAMA* article that starch blockers were necessarily ineffective. Prior research clearly showed that starch blockers were effective in test-tube experiments, or "in vitro." As a general rule, if actions occur in vitro, they will also probably occur within the human body, or "in vivo."

Therefore, Dr. DiMagno and his associates continued the research that had begun at the Howard Hughes Medical Institute, looking for ways to improve the extraction process. They needed to increase the amount of active starch-inhibition material in each dosage, and to eliminate all possible contaminants.

Major advances were made. A pure, much more active product was produced. In 1984, Dr. DiMagno, along with Drs. Peter Layer and Gerald Carlson, tested this new version of starch blockers against some of the old commercial formulas, and against crude bean extracts. The new Mayo Clinic formula was vastly more effective and proved quite capable in test tubes of inhibiting starch breakdown by human amylase.

This was the beginning of 15 years of starch blocker research by Mayo Clinic. Between 1984 and 1999, researchers there completed 13 studies and published all of them in peer-reviewed medical or scientific journals, including the *New England Journal of Medicine, Gastroenterology,* the *Mayo Clinic Proceedings, Pancreas,* and *Nutrition.*

The research of Dr. DiMagno and his colleagues laid the groundwork for all future investigation of starch blockers and became the "gold standard" against which later research was measured. Among the Mayo researchers' most significant determinations was, "We conclude that a purified amylase inhibitor is effective, and potentially beneficial in the treatment of diabetes mellitus."

Most of the Mayo Clinic research was aimed at investigating the use of starch blockers not against obesity but against diabetes. All of the results were promising. None of the research was definitive, however, as is generally the case when a new substance is tested against a deadly disease.

Mayo Clinic studies also tested the viability of wheat amylase inhibitors, but found that they were not strong enough to be effective in humans.

Mayo Clinic did do a small amount of research on weight loss, and found, not surprisingly, that because starch blockers inhibited starch digestion, they were also effective, in animal experiments, as a weight loss aid.

In Appendix C at the end of this book, you can find a listing of Mayo Clinic studies, with additional details and information on how to access these studies in their entirety. Appendix C also has details on 43 of the other most important studies.

Mayo Clinic studies gradually reignited interest in starch blockers among other members of the international biological research community, particularly in Japan. From 1992 until 2001, 11 separate studies were conducted at Kyushu University, Hokkaidō University of Sapporo, Osaka University, and at other Japanese universities and medical institutions. All were published in peer-reviewed, international medical journals.

Among the findings:

- Use of starch blockers heightened glucose stability in humans and reduced episodes of hypoglycemia.
- Starch blockers suppressed elevation of blood glucose immediately after people ate starch, thereby reducing triglycerides, free fatty acids, and total cholesterol.
- Starch blockers ameliorated various diabetes syndrome symptoms, including hypoglycemia.
- The hibiscus plant contains starch blockers, but the concentration of them is too low to be useful for stopping starch digestion in humans.
- Starch blockers create extra production of a substance called 3-hydroxybutyric acid, which has been shown in other studies to kill colon cancer cells.

Much of the Japanese research was aimed at improving the extraction methods for starch blockers. This research attracted virtually no interest from the general public, because it offered no immediate, practical application. However, it had a strong impact on the scientific community. As refinements were made in the process, starch blockers became increasingly effective and more financially feasible for commercial production. New studies on improved extraction methods proliferated around the world. Among the institutions that became involved were the University of California at San Diego, the University of Illinois, Canada's Institute for Biological Sciences, Brazil's University of Ponta Grossa, Northern Illinois University, and universities in Germany, France, and Scotland.

Despite this, major problems remained. By the mid-1990s, no institution had developed a refinement process that could deliver a highly potent version of starch blockers to the market at a price that most people could afford.

These problems were eventually solved by Pharmachem Laboratories of New Jersey. One of America's largest producers of bulk supplement products, this company is widely known for its emphasis on quality and purity and for its innovative techniques. At Pharmachem, Mitchell Skop, a research director and product developer, recognized the potential of starch blockers as a future weapon against diabetes, but also saw their immediate value as a weight management aid. Although this application seems stunningly obvious, particularly in light of starch blockers' brief but dramatic popularity as a weight control aid in 1982, it had been shunted aside by many researchers, who were more absorbed by starch blockers' potential for defeating diabetes. This degree of focus—some would say myopia—is not uncommon in science, particularly as it is practiced in academia. In major academic institutions, practicality often falls by the wayside.

Skop assigned a group of scientists, headed by Dilip Chokshi, to begin work on making a more potent, concentrated, and stable formula, one that would pass intact into the small intestine, where almost all starch digestion occurs. He also wanted to find ways to extract the formula using only purified water, and using only raw ingredients from non–genetically modified organisms that had been grown without pesticides and contained no heavy metals. In the language of laboratory production, the process had to be "durable," producing a substance that would survive in the digestive tract, and it had to be "reproducible," so that any other qualified laboratory in the world could produce it.

After several years, the biggest remaining problem was purity. It was difficult to remove 100% of the naturally occurring lectins in kidney beans, which cause mild digestive problems, such as bloating and gas. Eventually, the problem yielded to an elegantly simple solution: using smaller beans. It was discovered that the smallest of the northern white kidney beans, which contain the highest concentrations of starch blocker in the plant kingdom, have much lower concentrations of lectins then larger beans.

By 2000, Skop's research team was satisfied with their formula. "What we had produced," Skop later remarked, "was so different from the original formulas that it was no longer phaseolamin. However, everyone in the field of biological science was accustomed to the term 'phaseolamin,' so we just extrapolated from the common nomenclature and called it 'Phaseolamin 2250,' or 'Phase 2.'"

Phaseolamin 2250 was markedly stronger than Mayo Clinic's substance. It was more concentrated, more stable in the gastrointestinal tract, and was completely free of impurities.

Skop began to authorize testing of Phaseolamin 2250 (which we'll refer to hereinafter as Phase 2, for the sake of simplicity), as a weight loss aid in clinical studies.

One of the first tests was for safety. This test was performed in two segments by Dr. Radha Maheshwari, a scientist employed by the federal government's National Institutes of Health, although it was performed at a private research laboratory rather than in NIH facilities. In the first segment of the test, 160 rats were fed Phase 2 for 14 days, in varying dosages. The first group was fed 200 mg. of Phase 2 for every 5 kg. of their body weight—a very high dosage, in human terms. Four other groups were fed even higher amounts, with the fourth group receiving 25 times as much as the first group. The rats were monitored for adverse reactions, and after 14 days they were sacrificed. Their bodies were autopsied, their organs were examined, and their tissues were studied with electron microscopes. No abnormalities of any kind, nor any signs of toxicity, were discovered. In the next segment of the study, the rats were fed Phase 2 for 90 days instead of 14. Then the procedures were repeated with the same positive results. From this, it was concluded that Phase 2 was free of any toxic effects.

The next series of tests, performed at the University of Scranton, were double-blind, placebo-control studies that determined that Phase 2 blocked starch digestion in human volunteers. Four studies were done—under the direction of Professor Joe A. Vinson, Ph.D., of the department of chemistry—that proved conclusively that starch blockers inhibit starch digestion in humans.

In the first two studies, two groups of subjects were fed four slices of bread, and were then measured for blood glucose levels. The subjects in one of the groups took 1,500 mg. of starch blockers with the bread, and the other group took placebos. The group of subjects that had taken starch blockers experienced a noticeable flattening of the glycemic curve. Their blood glucose time curve—reflecting the amount of starch calories entering the bloodstream—was an average of 57% lower than that of subjects taking the placebo.

In a similar, subsequent trial, results were even better. Only 15% of the starch calories in the bread were absorbed.

In the third study, Dr. Vinson mixed powdered starch blocker into the mashed potatoes of a Hungry Man TV dinner containing steak, potatoes, green beans, mushrooms, gravy, and crumb cake.

In this study, the dosage of starch blocker was reduced by one-half, to 750 mg. It resulted in the blockage of only 28% of starch calories, which led Dr. Vinson to conclude that success appeared to be, to some degree, dose dependent. Dr. Vinson concluded that "an even more significant difference in starch absorption may occur if respondents are given a higher dose of Phase 2."

In 2001, at approximately the same time as the University of Scranton's series of studies, another study at the University of Illinois confirmed the ability of starch blockers to neutralize starch calories. Amylase activity was reduced by 50% to 75%, prompting researchers to conclude, "These results indicate that amylase inhibitor is effective in reducing amylase activity in vivo, and supports the hypothesis that an amylase inhibitor may reduce or delay carbohydrate absorption and glucose absorption."

Clearly, starch blockers could reduce starch calorie absorption. But could they help people reduce their levels of body fat? That question was answered by the remaining major studies, which dealt solely with weight loss.

The first of these studies was conducted in Norway by Parexel Medstat and was published in the *Journal of International Medical Research*. In a 12-week trial, 40 obese volunteers were randomly assigned administration of a starch blocker or a placebo. The subjects taking starch blockers were not required to adhere to a prudent diet, but they still averaged 7.4 pounds of weight loss, which was more than three times greater than the loss achieved by patients on placebo. Furthermore, it was determined that 85% of the weight loss in the starch blocker group was fat loss, rather than loss of muscle, which was a higher percentage than the norm.

The study was flawed in two ways, however, Subjects were mistakenly advised to take the starch blockers *after* meals, instead of before meals. This probably decreased the effectiveness of the starch blockers and may well have accounted for the fact that people in this study achieved less weight loss than people in subsequent studies. Furthermore, subjects were also given another weight management aid, *Garcinia cambogia,* which contains a substance, hydroxycitrate, that appears to be modestly helpful as a diet aid. The liability of taking the starch blockers too late in the meal probably hurt results more than the hydroxycitrate helped. However, these two factors still appear to have undermined the reliability of the study.

The next major study, by Italy's Pharmaceutical Development and Service, was conducted more carefully and achieved better results.

In this study, patients taking starch blockers lost an average of 3.9% of total body weight—or an average of 6.45 pounds—over 30 days, with no significant loss of muscle mass. This weight loss of approximately 1.5 pounds per week was composed almost solely of fat. This compared to a weight loss among patients on placebo of only one-half of 1%—about three-quarters of a pound for a 150-pound person over 30 days, or about one-sixth of a pound per week. In addition, the 30 patients taking starch blockers averaged, in just 30 days, a reduction of about 11% of all adipose tissue; a 3.44% reduction of waist measurement; a 1.39% reduction of hip circumference; and a 1.44% reduction of thigh circumference. Patients on the placebo achieved no significant reductions in body measurements.

In this study, patients were advised to take only one starch blocker tablet per day and were not encouraged to exercise. The patients were all at least 30 pounds overweight, were all healthy, and were age 20 to 45.

Afterwards, the chief researcher, Dr. R. Ballerini, concluded, "The study demonstrated the real capability of the considered product to determine in vivo weight loss through mass reduction, via reduced absorption, of complex carbohydrates."

The most well-conducted weight loss study to date, though, was performed in 2002 by Jay Udani, M.D., director of the Integrative Medicine Program at Northridge Hospital (a UCLA affiliate).

In his study, 50 patients, all under age 50, with body mass indexes of 30 to 35 (indicating obesity), were given either 1,500 mg. of the Phase 2 formula up to twice a day, or a placebo, to be ingested with starchy meals. The study was randomized and double-blind, and lasted for eight weeks.

The subjects were advised to eat daily diets that contained a moderate amount of carbohydrates—up to 200 grams, or 800 calories. They were also advised to eat diets that were relatively low in fat and relatively high in fiber.

The primary factor the study examined was weight loss. The secondary factors were the impact of starch blockers on triglycerides and waist measurements. In addition, Dr. Udani monitored patients for a subjective sense of well-being.

The results, made available especially for this book by Dr. Udani, are dramatic and compelling. In this book, however, no statistical analysis has been applied, as would be the style in medical journal articles.

The most relevant finding in the study was that the patients taking starch blockers lost an average of approximately four pounds over the course of the study, compared to an average of one and one-half pounds lost by the patients on placebo. This is a difference of approximately 230%.

The amount of weight lost was less than that lost by subjects in the study by Dr. Ballerini, but this degree of variation is not unusual in studies such as these, in which subjects' caloric intake is self-determined and can vary greatly. Even though Dr. Udani recommended that his subjects eat a low-fat, high-fiber diet that was moderate in carbs, he had no control over their adherence to the guidelines. It is predictable in this kind of a study that many subjects will stray from the guidelines and not report their indulgences, perhaps because of embarrassment or simply a lack of awareness of their caloric intake. However, this variance could be expected equally from both the starch blocker group and the placebo group, so a sensible way to accurately interpret the outcome is to primarily compare the results of the two groups. In this comparison, the starch blocker group obviously fared far better than the control group at losing weight.

The starch blocker group was also more successful at losing inches. By eight weeks, they had lost an average of slightly more than one and one-half inches from their waists, which was 40% more than the average of the control group.

Some of the most revealing data came from objective measurements of triglycerides. Blood levels of triglycerides, which are the form in which fats are stored in the body, went down dramatically among starch blocker users, averaging a drop of 26 mg. per deciliter. Among the control group, triglycerides stayed at the same general plateau, dropping only 7 mg. per deciliter. Thus, the starch blocker group had a 370% better decline than the control group.

There was also a difference in how much better the starch blocker group felt, compared to the control group. This is critically important, because how people feel in a weight management program is arguably the best predictor of how well they will succeed. Even if they're doing well by objective measurements—losing weight and inches and lowering their blood fat levels—they still usually don't succeed in the long run unless they're also feeling good. The starch blocker group felt better. They experienced a trend toward improvement in energy, even though the starch blocker is not a stimulant. This is a primary factor in keeping weight from creeping back on. Virtually no one can endure a painful diet forever.

Another revealing aspect of the study results was the analysis of the top performers. Among the group of starch blocker users, the five leading weight losers lost 18 pounds, 17 pounds, 10.5 pounds, 7 pounds, and 6.5 pounds (a combined total of 59 pounds). Among the control group, the five leading weight losers lost 6 pounds, 6 pounds, 5 pounds, 4.5 pounds, and 3 pounds (a combined total of 24.5 pounds). "These are the results that are possible," Dr. Udani noted, "though not typical."

At the conclusion of this study, Dr. Udani was impressed. "Apparently, the starch blocker substance, when used with daily ingestion of up to 200 grams of carbohydrate, contributed to persistent and steady weight loss," he said. "It appears to have had an effect on carbohydrate management by the body, as indicated by the triglyceride indexes." These were very positive trends.

"In my opinion," said Dr. Udani, "the ideal way to lose weight is slowly and consistently, at the rate of approximately one-half to one pound per week. People using this substance were able to approximate that goal, while still eating a nutritious and well-balanced diet, which included reasonable amounts of carbohydrates.

"The primary reason most people appear to be unable to lose

weight and maintain that weight loss over the long term," he said, "is because of general dissatisfaction with weight management diets. It's my opinion, though, that people will be able to stick with the starch blocker weight management approach, and thereby be able to lose a significant amount of weight and keep it off over an extended period of time."

Dr. Udani did not recommend exercise to the people in his study because he wanted to determine if use of starch blockers alone resulted in weight loss. However, he has stated, "I believe that if people do add a prudent regimen of exercise to this protocol, they may be able to achieve a weight loss goal of approximately one pound per week, and maintain this rate of weight loss as they work toward their ideal goal weights."

THE FUTURE

It appears as if the future is bright for further research on starch blockers. The obvious opportunity is for their use against diabetes. However, starch blockers may also prove to be helpful in controlling at least two types of cancer associated with the digestive tract.

The first is colon cancer. It has long been known that increased digestive fiber is very helpful for preventing colon cancer. The presumed mechanism of action for this protection is decreased bowel transit time for digested food. The longer digested food remains in the colon, the more damage it is believed to do. Starch blockers create an effect that is similar to the ingestion of dietary fiber. By causing starch to remain in whole-molecule form, starch blockers effectively increase the fibrous texture of starch. In fact, many people have noticed that when they take starch blockers, it has somewhat the same effect upon their systems of elimination as does eating more fiber. Some people who have long suffered from chronic constipation have noticed improvement when they began taking starch blockers.

Thus, this bulking effect may prove to exert colon cancer benefits similar to those created by the bulking action of fiber.

In addition, there's a relatively new theory about why fiber helps prevent colon cancer. According to it, fiber helps by mildly increasing fermentation in the bowel, which produces the chemical butyric acid. Recently, it was discovered that butyric acid inhibits growth of colon cancer cells. It helps stop them from growing by regulating a substance called epidermal growth factor, and also by regulating estrogen receptors.

Starch blockers also mildly increase fermentation in the bowel, increasing production of butyric acid. Theoretically, this increase in butyric acid may help control colon cancer cell growth.

Therefore, starch blockers may one day prove to be a helpful ally against colon cancer, which is one of the leading causes of cancer death among men and women combined.

Another promising benefit that may come from starch blockers is help in preventing pancreatic cancer. In an article last year in the *Journal of the National Cancer Institute,* it was revealed that a study at Boston's Brigham and Women's Hospital of 89,000 women showed that women who ate high amounts of starch and didn't exercise regularly were 250% more likely than others to contract pancreatic cancer, a form of cancer that is virtually incurable. Researchers examined starch intake as a factor in pancreatic cancer because previous research had shown that when an excessive amount of insulin is present in the pancreas, it enhances cancer cell growth in that organ. Starchy foods, as you know, are notorious for increasing insulin levels.

The pancreas, of course, is also where the starch-digesting enzyme alpha amylase is produced. Therefore, it's also possible that excessive starch intake simply exhausts the pancreas and makes it more vulnerable to disease.

At this point, these theories are merely speculative. However, twenty years ago, virtually *everything* about starch blockers was considered speculative.

Thus far, starch blockers have lived up to the potential they promised back in 1973, when Howard Hughes first saw an article about rats starving to death in Venezuela.

Who can fully predict what promise they hold for the future?

PART TWO

THE STRATEGY'S THREE STEPS

FOUR

STEP ONE: REDISTRIBUTING CALORIES

The Starch Blocker Diet

My patient knew something few in the world knew, and it had put a gleam in his eye.

He was a professor at UCLA, and for the past several days, word had been leaking out of the UCLA School of Medicine that results of a just-completed clinical trial were promising to change the field of weight management forever. The clinical trial was Dr. Jay Udani's study on starch blockers.

The professor's eager anticipation of this breakthrough was practically palpable, probably because he had a serious weight problem. Fat was climbing out of his collar, and his face was florid with the excessive circulation that obese people require, even while inactive.

"Have you heard about starch neutralizers?" he asked.

"Starch blockers? I have. I've been recommending them to a number of patients recently."

"I want some." Simple as that. He was sold. But I wanted him to think about it. People who rush into things rarely succeed.

"Why? What have *you* heard?" I asked.

"I heard you can eat virtually anything, and still lose significant adipose tissue."

"That's not true."

"I heard you don't have to exercise."

"Not true, either."

"Dessert at every meal?"

I shook my head.

"Then what's the big deal?"

"The big deal is that they level the playing field."

"Explain that."

"Do you eat excessively?" I asked him.

He looked reflective, and I felt he was trying to give me an honest answer.

"I probably do eat more than I should. But I eat about the same as my kids and my wife, and they're not overweight. I don't eat enough to deserve to look like this." He looked down at his body, then down at the floor.

"I'll take your word for it," I said. "That's more common than you might think. A number of studies—good, peer-reviewed ones— have shown that a high percentage of overweight people eat moderately. Many of them eat less than thin people."

He looked up. The gleam was back. "That's me."

"That's a lot of people. Life isn't fair, and neither is the human metabolism. At least seventy-five percent of all overweight people have significantly abnormal carbohydrate metabolisms, and it sounds as if you're probably one of them. For people like you, the playing field isn't level. It's tilted against you. But starch blockers level the field by removing abnormal starch metabolism from the equation of weight management. They'll make your carbohydrate metabolism function more like the carb metabolism of a thin person. But you'll have to *eat* like a thin person. And exercise, too."

"So they're not a panacea."

"By no means."

He was an intelligent man, and actually seemed relieved to land back in reality. Smart people know that when something sounds too good to be true, it usually is.

"So how does one start?" he asked. "By taking the pills?"

"No. You start by changing your diet."

In the world of weight management, everything starts with dietary change. Always has. Always will.

CALORIC SHIFTING

Right now, you may be waiting for the proverbial ax to fall. This is usually the part of the diet book where the doctor tells you about all the calories you need to cut.

Not this time. This is different.

The starch blocker diet consists primarily of *shifting* calories, not eliminating them. Eliminating them is the starch blocker's job.

Essentially, you need to shift your diet away from excessive fats and sugars, and compensate for those lost calories by consuming more starch and more protein. The starch blocker will then neutralize the starch calories, leaving you with a far lower net caloric intake than before. When that happens, your body, deprived of the easy-burning carbs, will start burning body fat.

The chart below outlines a basic eating plan for starting the starch blocker diet that will work with great effectiveness for almost all people. This plan is designed to create a moderate, steady weight loss of about 1.5 to 2 pounds per week. This degree of weight loss (or slightly more—up to about 3 pounds) is approximately as much as most people can achieve without triggering the starvation effect of caloric hoarding, which is responsible for much of the rebound weight gain that typically occurs following an excessive, crash diet. This amount of weight loss per week is also about as much as most people can lose without starting to consume their own muscle tissues, including the muscle tissues of the vital organs, such as the heart. If you lose 2 to 3 pounds (or less) per week, your weight loss will almost certainly be composed of a very high percentage of body fat. The only exception to this will be in the very beginning of the diet, when the loss of excess water weight may also occur.

The Starch Blocker Diet
Before Caloric Neutralization

Starch: 45% of the diet

Sugars: 12% of the diet

Fat: 15% of the diet

Protein: 28% of the diet

At first glance, you might be thinking, "Hold on! When I add the starch and sugar together to determine the total carb intake, 57% of this diet is carbohydrates. That's the same old high-carb diet that's been such a catastrophe!"

However, *if you use starch blockers with the starch blocker diet,* it will dramatically alter the ratios of the various food components, because starch blockers will neutralize approximately 75% of all starch calories, resulting in the following changes.

The Starch Blocker Diet
Adjusted for Starch Calorie Neutralization

Starch: 17% of the diet

Sugars: 18% of the diet

Fat: 22% of the diet

Protein: 43% of the diet

Let's take a look at how these ratios stack up in terms of calories. If you were eating a 2,500 calorie per day diet, which is approximately average for most normal-size, relatively active people, your caloric intake would look like this, *before* taking starch blockers:

The Starch Blocker Diet Expressed in Calories
Before Caloric Neutralization

Starch:	1,125	calories per day
Sugars:	300	calories per day
Fat:	375	calories per day
Protein:	700	calories per day
Total:	2,500	calories per day

This eating plan is practical, sensible, and not particularly difficult. Here's a general idea of what it might contain.

- **Breakfast** could be pancakes with butter and syrup, accompanied by orange juice and milk, followed by a midmorning snack of banana bread topped with low-fat cream cheese, and tea.
- **Lunch** could consist of a hearty vegetable soup, a turkey sandwich, a side order of potato salad, and some braised asparagus. Lunch could be followed with a low-calorie dessert, or with a midafternoon snack of a piece of fruit.
- **Dinner** could be a chicken breast sautéed in olive oil and garlic, along with a baked potato, an ear of corn on the cob, a tomato and lettuce salad with vinaigrette dressing, and a dinner roll with butter. You could also have a glass of wine before dinner, or perhaps a beer. A snack before bed could be a bowl of popcorn, with a glass of iced fruit juice.

Obviously, this isn't a starvation diet. But for most average-size people, it's not a weight loss diet, either.

However, when you take starch blockers with this general eating plan, it *does* become a weight loss diet. Here's how it will look in terms of calories when you accompany your meals with starch blockers.

The Starch Blocker Diet
Adjusted for Starch Calorie Neutralization
Expressed in Calories

Starch:	281	calories per day
Sugars:	300	calories per day
Fat:	375	calories per day
Protein:	700	calories per day
Total:	1,656	calories per day

As you can see, the calories from sugars, fat, and protein remain the same, but the calories from starch are drastically reduced—by 75%. This 75% reduction accounts for a decrease in total starch calories from 1,125 to just 281. That's a difference of 844 calories per day, or a whopping 5,908 calories per week.

Approximately 3,500 dietary calories are required to create one pound of body fat, and it requires the same number of calories to be avoided or burned through exercise—or neutralized—to create the *loss* of one pound of body fat. Therefore, when you eliminate 5,908 calories per week, through neutralization of starch calories, you can expect to lose approximately 1.5 pounds of body fat per week (through diet alone, without exercise).

This is a safe and sane amount of fat loss to achieve each week. And remember—it is *fat* loss you're striving for, not weight loss. Weight loss can include the loss of muscle tissue, which is very harmful. Your muscles help you look fit and attractive, and are of obvious value in helping you maintain your exercise program. In addition, muscles burn fat much more efficiently than nonmuscle tissues, such as body fat. Furthermore, when muscle cells are lost through dieting, they tend to be primarily replaced by fat cells during any period of rebound weight gain.

This amount of weight loss can also be accompanied by water weight loss, which many diet gurus have traditionally dismissed as insignificant. I don't necessarily agree with that. As my coauthor, Cameron Stauth, demonstrated in his award-winning book *The False Fat Diet,* excessive water weight can persist *perpetually,* bloating people with a "false fat" that is just as uncomfortable, unattractive, and almost as unhealthy as adipose tissue, or true fat. This perpetual water weight gain mostly occurs because of allergylike food reactions, which we'll discuss later in this chapter. However, it also occurs simply because of excessive intake of carbohydrates, which require water for storage.

The loss of this false fat will add to the amount of weight that you lose, especially during the first few weeks of the strategy.

The other major factor that will boost your fat loss when you participate in the strategy is, of course, exercise. One hour of moderate exercise burns approximately 500 calories, so if you exercise an hour every day, you can expect to burn about 3,500 extra calories per week. This should account for one more pound of fat loss each week. Of course, it probably won't cause one pound of *weight* loss, because your exercise will add weight to your muscles. For example, Cameron Stauth noted that when he initially began taking starch blockers, he lost about 20 pounds of weight, but when his body fat was measured, it became clear that he'd lost approximately 30 pounds of fat, and had gained almost 10 pounds of muscle.

Therefore, we believe it's wise for strategists to abandon the general public's common fixation upon scale weight and to focus instead upon body fat percentage, which we'll show you how to calculate in Chapter Eight.

Another way to gauge your success is to monitor your increase in fitness, with simple tests of speed, endurance, and strength. Fitness is fantastic. In many ways, it's more important than thinness. People who are fit, even if they're carrying a couple of extra pounds, are almost always more healthy and attractive than people who are merely thin, but not fit.

An even easier way to measure your progress is just to look in the mirror. If you like what you see, you're succeeding.

If you don't think you're losing fat fast enough, though, be patient. Some people are tempted to eat almost all starch and to block every bit of it, but it's not at all smart to totally avoid fats and proteins. The body requires balance in its intake of nutrients. Without sufficient balance, you'll become weak and ill.

If you've been on other popular diets, you know that even the most extreme of these still require a degree of balance among each of the three primary food categories. For example, most low-carbohydrate diets recommend that you eat about 40% of your diet as protein, 30% as carbohydrates, and 30% as fats. Even the most rigid low-fat diets recommend that you eat about 10% to 20% of your diet as protein, 60% to 70% as carbohydrates, and 10% to 20% as fats.

Compare these ratios to the starch blocker diet ratios. On our plan, if you combine the sugars and starch as carbs, the ratios are: 43% protein, 22% fat, and 35% carbohydrates (when starch blockers are taken with meals). Therefore, compared to the other diets, the starch blocker diet is moderate.

However, the starch blocker diet is much closer to the low-carb diets than the high-carb diets. Because of its low-carb content, the starch blocker diet doesn't trigger insulin instability.

Even though the starch blocker diet is low in carbs, though, it's *still low in fat*. That's absolutely unique. Virtually all of the current, popular low-carb diets are *much* higher in fat than the starch blocker diet. These low-carb diets require relatively high consumption of fat mainly in order to compensate for the avoidance of carb calories, and thus keep people from being hungry. For people using the strategy, though, carb calorie elimination is the job of the starch blocker, *not* the dieter. The starch blocker neutralizes these harmful, fast-burning carb calories after they're consumed. Consuming these calories, however, keeps people from being hungry and makes them far less dependent upon fat calories for fighting hunger. We'll tell you all about hunger—and how to avoid it—in the next chapter.

The advent of low-carb diets has had a positive effect upon American eating habits. These diets have helped people realize that high carb consumption is the worst culprit in America's current epidemic of diabetes caused by obesity, or "diabesity." However, clinical evidence tends to indicate that the starch blocker diet can be even *more* effective than most low-carb diets against diabesity, for two reasons. First, it's easier to follow than the traditional low-carb diets. Second, it's lower in fat.

Therefore, if you've been successful on low-carb diets in the past, the starch blocker diet may be perfect for you. It makes a low-carb diet much more enjoyable and easier to sustain. Furthermore, when you add starchy foods to a low-carb diet, but neutralize these foods' starch calories, you reap a huge bonus of extra vitamins, minerals, and fiber.

You may have noticed that the starch blocker diet has a higher percentage of protein than other low-carb diets. One simple reason for this is that the starch blocker diet can *afford* to pile on the protein calories, due to the reduction of starch calories caused by the starch blocker.

Protein is a superb foodstuff. It's satisfying, slow-burning, and uniquely rich in the nutrients the body needs to repair itself. However, most diets just can't afford to include as much protein as we recommend, simply because it would add too many calories to regimes already bloated with starch calories.

Caloric neutralization is the beauty of this strategy! It allows people to shift their dietary intake to the nutrients they really need, without adding excess net calories.

Now let's take a closer look at each of the three basic components of your diet—protein, fat, and carbohydrates—and see how each will fit into your new starch blocker diet.

PROTEIN: THE BODY BUILDER

Protein is the only substance that rebuilds the body. The *only* one.

Other nutrients, such as vitamins, minerals, and essential fatty acids, help protein rebuild the body and are necessary for biological function, but protein alone provides the building blocks of life. These building blocks—the amino acids that combine to form protein—repair and replace millions of cells throughout your body every day. The amino acids in protein form your muscles, skin, bone, tissues, teeth, organs, hair—in short, your entire body.

Found primarily in meat, eggs, poultry, fish, nuts, dairy products, and some plant foods (particularly soy products and beans), protein is also a fine source of food energy, otherwise known as calories. Calories from high-protein foods are the exact opposite of the empty calories that compose sugars and refined starches. High-protein foods are loaded not only with amino acids, but also with vitamins, minerals, and enzymes. They are the ultimate "full" calorie.

When you don't get enough protein, your body literally begins to fall apart. Your hair can become thin, or fall out. Your skin can age prematurely, your eyes can become weak, and many necessary biological functions can cease. Your muscles, in particular, can become atrophied and flaccid from protein deprivation as muscle tissue dissolves.

The loss of muscle tissue is common among dieters, and it is a terrible, ironic waste of these dieters' hard effort and denial. Without enough dietary protein, this loss of muscle can be hard to avoid, since muscle makes up approximately one-half of all body weight.

Overweight people sometimes think they don't have very much muscle, but that's not true. They frequently have more muscle, by weight, than thin people, simply because it requires a lot of muscle for them to carry around their excess weight.

Protein also feeds the muscles that compose your internal organs, such as those of your heart, lungs, liver, and kidneys, which are the most metabolically active tissues in your body. In addition, the amino acids that form protein are used to create neurotransmitters, blood cells, immune system cells, and hormones.

The minimum amount of protein you need depends upon how active you are. Inactive people need less, mostly because their muscles are consuming less protein for repair and rebuilding. To figure out your own minimum protein needs, use one of the following equations:

MINIMUM PROTEIN NEEDS

- *Inactive People.* Divide your weight by 2. This number is equal to the number of protein grams you need per day. To figure the minimum number of protein *calories* you need per day, multiply the grams by 4.
- *Active People.* Your weight is the same number as the minimum number of protein grams you need per day. To figure the minimum number of protein *calories* you need per day, multiply the grams by 4.

Using these formulas, you can see that a 150-pound, inactive person would need a minimum of 75 grams of protein per day (300 calories), and an active 150-pound person would need at least 150 grams (600 calories).

Thus, some of the popular diets—particularly the low-fat, high-carb diets—are dangerously close to protein deficiency. A 2,500-calorie-per-day diet that's only 10% protein, for example, would provide only 250 calories. For most people, this isn't enough. It tends to make people feel weak and lethargic, and even causes mental lassitude, since protein is used to manufacture the brain's neurotransmitters. Over an extended period of time, this protein deprivation can contribute to illness and degeneration.

Keep in mind, too, that these are *minimum* protein requirements, not optimal requirements.

We believe that for optimal function, protein intake should be in the range of 40% of the total diet (or about 700 calories for a 150-pound, active person).

Excessive protein intake can be harmful, though. It's particularly stressful on the kidneys, which must remove all excess protein from the body. Therefore, it's important to not get too much of a good thing. Protein intake of about 40% of the diet should be safe for almost all normally healthy people. Anything in excess of 75% to 85% could be dangerous.

FAT: YOUR POTENTIAL FOE

When people do not succeed using the starch blocker strategy—and not all people do—it is most often because they eat too much fat. These days, when the general trend in nutritional science is to focus on the damage done by excessive carbohydrate intake, it's easy for many people to overlook the harm done by dietary fat. Also, there's a tendency for people to think that most Americans aren't currently consuming very much fat, because consumption has dropped over the last 10 to 15 years from an average of 40% of the diet to a current average of 34% of the diet. This decrease is a good thing, but what rarely gets mentioned is that between 1910 and 1980, consumption of fat *increased* by almost 50%. Therefore, from a broader historical perspective, people are still eating more fat than their ancestors ate.

One reason people are eating more fat these days is because beef, a primary source of dietary fat, is significantly higher in fat than it used to be. The free-range beef eaten in the early 1900s was about 3% to 7% fat, while today's prime feedlot cattle average about 30% fat (almost 1,700 calories per pound).

Ironically, today's cattle have been made this fat by widespread use among farmers of the U.S. Department of Agriculture's "Feedlot Guidelines," which call for feeding cattle 61% carbohydrates (mostly starch), 25% fat, and 14% protein. These ratios are very similar to those recommended in the recently replaced USDA food guidelines for *people*. This prompted one prominent academician from the Harvard School of Public Health to remark recently that the American diet has become "the great American feedlot."

An even bigger reason for America's current overconsumption of fat, though, is the trend toward eating more meals in restaurants. About 20% of all meals are now eaten in restaurants—most often, fast-food restaurants. With some exceptions, fast food is notoriously high in fat. Look at these high amounts of fat calories in popular fast foods:

Fat Calories
In Popular Fast Foods

Taco Bell Bellgrande Nachos	317 fat calories
Burger King Scrambled Egg Platter with Sausage	468 fat calories
McDonald's Big Mac	291 fat calories
McDonald's Medium Fries	154 fat calories
Taco Bell Taco, light	259 fat calories
KFC Extra Crispy Breast	213 fat calories

Just one serving of any of these fast foods uses up most, or all, of the fat calories that we recommend for an entire day. Therefore, if you insist on eating fast foods on the starch blocker diet, scan the calorie charts that are posted in the restaurants and make a wise choice, such as a grilled chicken breast sandwich with no mayonnaise. This selection only has 28 fat calories. Then, if you block most of the 152 starch calories from the bun of the chicken sandwich, you're left with a high-protein, low-calorie lunch.

Besides strictly limiting fat calories, you should also pay careful attention to the *type* of fat you're eating. There are good fats and bad fats, even though *all* fats are high in calories—9 calories per gram, compared to 4 calories per gram for carbs and protein. Oils, which are just liquid fat, are also 9 calories per gram. However, despite the high calories in fat, some fats and oils can actually help you lose weight. These good fats are the essential fatty acids, or EFAs, including the omega-3 oils. EFAs are absolutely essential for life; in effect, they are the "vitamins" of the fat world. Your body can't produce them, and without them, you would die. They come primarily from nuts and seeds, such vegetables as olives and avocados, deep-water ocean fish (such as salmon, tuna, and halibut), some fruits, and to a lesser extent, meat and poultry.

EFAs are used by the body to produce energy within cells, and if they are eaten in relatively high amounts—composing about 15% of all caloric intake—they significantly increase the metabolic rate and spur the burning of body fat. We recommend that you try to derive about half your fat intake from EFAs. Among the best ways to do this is to use olive oil as your primary oil for cooking and salad dressing, to eat fish at least a couple of times per week, and to snack on nuts instead of starchy foods.

EFAs are so effective at increasing metabolic rate that some of them are sold in capsules as diet supplements. For example, in a recent study at the University of Wisconsin, the EFA linoleic acid was used as a weight loss supplement, along with a low-calorie diet, and helped subjects to lose an average of approximately 20% of their body fat. This weight loss was significantly better than that of a control group that didn't take linoleic acid, but was still on a low-calorie diet.

Furthermore, when people taking linoleic acid regain weight after returning to their normal diets, they tend to regain relatively more *muscle* and less *fat*. In the Wisconsin study, when some of the subjects taking linoleic acid regained weight, their weight was an average of 55% lean muscle mass and 45% fat, compared to 75% lean muscle and 25% fat in the control group of people who were not taking linoleic acid.

One of the main reasons why EFAs are the healthiest type of fat is that they are not saturated with hydrogen atoms, which makes fat molecules stick together. When fats are full of hydrogen atoms, they are thick and sticky, like lard and shortening. They don't melt at room temperature, and they don't naturally dissolve in the body. Instead, they clump together on blood vessel walls, narrowing the paths of blood flow and hardening the walls of blood vessels. In addition, these fats cause blood cells to clump together. The net result, of course, is cardiovascular disease, the leading cause of death in America.

Not all of the fat that ends up in the bloodstream comes from dietary fat, though. Much of it simply comes from overeating—including eating too much starch. When this happens, the body converts the extra calories to fat, and some of it ends up in the bloodstream.

Saturated fats, though, are harmful to more than just the cardiovascular system. They enter every cell in the body, including the brain cells, thickening the walls of these cells. When cell walls get too thick, cells have a hard time letting nutrients in and getting toxins out. They become damaged and can begin to die.

All EFAs are unsaturated and so are some other common oils. The molecules of unsaturated fats are not packed tightly together, so they don't cause nearly as much thickening and hardening of blood vessel walls and cell walls as saturated fats. They also don't raise cholesterol levels in the blood.

There are two types of unsaturated fats—monounsaturated and polyunsaturated. Monounsaturated fats are the least "packed together," so they're the healthiest.

Here are some unsaturated fats, ranked from best to worst. Of these, only olive oil and canola oil are monounsaturated, and the rest are polyunsaturated.

1. Virgin olive oil (monounsaturated)

2. Canola oil (monounsaturated)

3. Peanut oil

4. Soybean oil

5. Corn oil

6. Sunflower oil

7. Safflower oil

There's one type of fat, though, that's *really* a disaster. It's even worse than the other saturated fats—and it happens to be the single most popular form of fat in America. That fat is the hydrogenated trans-fatty acid found in foods such as margarine. Margarine, unfortunately, is the country's leading single source of fat, accounting for more dietary fat than even beef.

Hydrogenated fats are oils that have been artificially bombarded with hydrogen atoms in order to make them solid. This process gives margarine and other hydrogenated products a nice texture, but in terms of health, it's a catastrophe. One large study, for example, showed that women who ate four or more teaspoons of margarine every day had a 66% higher incidence of cardiovascular disease than women who rarely ate margarine.

Hydrogenated fats are death waiting to happen. When you want butter, eat butter—not margarine—even though some margarines are less fattening than butter. To save calories, use whipped butter.

You may have noticed that in much of this section on fats, we've focused more on health than upon weight loss. There's a reason. Health is *everything*. Weight management is just a part of it. *If you just strive for thin, you'll never win.* But if you strive for vibrant health, thin will follow, as a natural consequence.

One last word about the danger of eating too much fat. Whenever you eat something, your body spends energy converting that food into useful energy. When you eat carbs and protein, researchers believe that you burn up to 20% of the total calories in those foods as you convert them into energy. But fat converts into energy too easily. It only requires about 3% of its calories for conversion. Therefore, lots of fat calories are left, and many of them can end up as body fat.

Don't destroy your starch blocker diet by eating too much fat. It's easy to do. Check the calorie list in Chapter Eight whenever you're tempted to have a high-fat food. When you see how fattening these foods can be, you might not be so tempted.

CARBOHYDRATES: KNOW YOUR ENEMY

Here's a quiz to take. Be painfully honest in your responses. If you aren't, you won't learn how to help yourself with the starch blocker strategy.

Give yourself one point if the following characterizations are sometimes true or if they describe you moderately well; two points if they are often true or describe you quite well; and three points if they're virtually always true and describe you perfectly.

The Carb Quiz

1. My fat storage is more in my abdomen than my hips or thighs.

2. Dinner doesn't feel complete without dessert.

3. Right after I eat sweets or something very high in starch, such as a big dinner roll, I feel satisfied and content.

4. I tend to get hungry about an hour or two after meals.

5. I really enjoy caffeinated drinks, and feel great after a cappuccino or a diet cola.

6. I love Italian food and Chinese food, probably even more than rich French food, or high-fat American home cooking.

7. It makes me feel good to chew gum, or to have a mint or a piece of hard candy in my mouth.

8. For snacks, I would usually prefer chips or a bagel over nuts or an apple.

9. I drink diet soft drinks almost every day to cut back on calories.

10. High-fat, nonsweet foods such as beef or butter are good, but they're not my weakness.

11. High-fat, sweet foods, such as rich desserts, are extremely tempting to me, even though I know they're too fattening.

12. Diabetes runs in my family.

13. When I get hungry before a meal, I'm pretty uncomfortable, and really need to eat.

14. I have to watch myself, or I'll drink more alcohol than I really should.

15. I've never stayed at my ideal weight for more than about a year.

16. I take a serotonin-influencing antidepressant, such as Paxil, Zoloft, or Prozac.

17. Hunger definitely affects my mood. When I'm hungry, I get irritable, and sometimes feel spaced-out.

18. When I start eating ice cream, cookies, or other favorite sweets, it's hard to stop, and I sometimes eat more than I'd planned to.

19. When I've tried low-carb diets, I've felt good, but I really missed my high-carb foods.

20. I think I gain weight more easily than most people.

21. It seems to me as if my metabolism has really changed for the worse as I've gotten older. I have to eat less and exercise more just to keep from gaining.

22. I sometimes wake up at night feeling hungry.

23. If I don't get lunch on time, it's very hard to work.

24. Several times almost every day, I think about food while I work.

25. I seem to have less willpower about eating than I do about other aspects of my life.

This is an easy quiz to flunk.

It determines your general sensitivity to carbohydrates, and *most* people are overly sensitive to carbohydrates—especially overweight people.

Here's the good news, though. The worse you score on this test, the more likely you'll be to benefit greatly from starch blockers. If you are highly sensitive to carbs, starch blockers are exactly what you need.

Scoring Your Quiz

Score

3–8   **Excellent score.** Starch blockers might not help much, because your carb metabolism functions well.

9–12   **You have a few problems with carbs,** but are basically in control of them. However, you might benefit from a starch blocker once a day, or every other day, to prevent future problems.

13–25   **Possible trouble.** You probably need to restrict sweets and neutralize most of the starch you eat in order to have the same metabolic advantages of a person with a healthy carb metabolism.

26–50   **Be wary.** Get busy. You have significant dysfunction of carb metabolism and are probably already suffering from hypoglycemia or hyperglycemia. You need to limit sugar intake and take starch blockers to restore healthy carb metabolism.

50 or over **You're in trouble,** and you should deal with it immediately. You probably already suffer from Syndrome X, or are headed for it. If you don't do something to prevent it, diabetes is a very realistic possibility. Starch blockers will probably improve your quality of life almost immediately.

Unfortunately, in our current carb-obsessed culture, a score of 25 to 50 is not at all uncommon. It's not cause for alarm. But it is cause for action.

Take this quiz again after you've been using the strategy for a couple of months. If you're like most people, your score will improve considerably. Use of starch blockers has a tremendously positive impact upon abnormal carb metabolism and should help restore yours to the healthy function you may have experienced when you were much younger.

If you scored poorly on this quiz, it's important for you to be vigilant about following the starch blocker strategy. Take starch blockers with practically every starchy meal and snack. Limit your sugar intake aggressively. Exercise regularly. Assert your emotional power over food. And when you eat starchy foods, eat the *right* starchy foods.

The right starchy foods are those that are minimally processed, or not processed at all. When starchy foods are processed, or refined, they can rush into the bloodstream as quickly as pure sugar—sometimes even *more* quickly. The processing destroys factors that slow down digestion, such as fiber and large starch granules.

Think of eating highly refined starches as drinking alcohol on an empty stomach. If you've ever had a couple of drinks without eating something first, you know that alcohol on an empty stomach hits the system hard. So does fast-burning, highly refined starch. Think of eating *unrefined* starches as drinking on a *full* stomach.

Some people who take starch blockers think that it doesn't matter much if the starchy foods they eat are highly processed, since the starch calories from these foods will be blocked, anyway. But they're overlooking an important detail. Not *all* the starch calories get blocked. About 25% of them slip past the starch blocker, and you want that 25% to consist of slow-burning starchy foods, not fast-burning starchy foods.

The rating of how fast various carbs burn is called the glycemic index. When you study more about the glycemic index in Chapter Eight, you'll get some surprises. The biggest surprise, for most people, is that many highly refined starchy foods sprint into the bloodstream just as fast as pure sucrose, or white sugar. Look at the high glycemic indexes of the following foods, some of which you probably thought were healthy. Pure sugar has a glycemic index of 65, but the index of every one of these foods is *even higher*.

Fast-Burning Starchy Foods
(compared to white sugar, with an index of 65)

Starchy Food	Glycemic Index
Rice Krispies	82
Bagel	72
Rye bread	76
Waffles	76
Parsnips	97
Baked potato, without skin	93
Corn chips	72
Pretzels	83

(For more on glycemic indexes, see Chapter Eight.)

Of course, the glycemic index of various foods is less important to strategists than to anyone else on any other kind of diet, since starch blockers do eliminate 75% of starch calories. Even so, never forget about the 25% of all starch calories that do evade the starch blockade. For complete success, you should still try to eat foods with a low glycemic index. A low index is about 30 to 50.

Several factors, most of which are related to the refining process, influence a food's glycemic index. One is cooking. When starchy foods are cooked, it makes them easier to digest and raises their glycemic index. Therefore, raw foods are generally preferable. Another factor is the particle size of the food. When starchy foods such as grains are milled, the crushing process reduces the size of the starchy food particles and makes them burn more easily. That's why foods from highly processed grains, such as white bread, have dangerously high indexes. The presence of fat also slows absorption, and reduces the glycemic index of foods that are high in both carbs and fat, such as ice cream. However, fat adds its own calories, so it doesn't confer much of an advantage.

Another important factor that increases glycemic index is the abundant presence of a substance called amylopectin, which makes starch easier to digest. Wheat flour, for example, is rich in amylopectin and therefore burns more quickly than starchy foods that are low in amylopectin, such as long-grain rice, and beans.

The final—and most important—factor that influences glycemic index is fiber. Fiber can drastically slow the burning of starch, because it's a tough substance that's hard to digest, and is often impossible to fully digest. However, fiber doesn't really help if it's been pulverized in the refining process. For example, many brands of bran flakes are high in fiber, but that fiber has been finely ground during the processing of the cereals, seriously harming its ability to slow down starch digestion. Similarly, some whole wheat breads have a glycemic index that's only slightly better than that of white bread.

Even so, many high-fiber foods survive the milling process with their fibers mostly intact, and therefore have markedly lower indexes. Kellogg's All-Bran with Extra Fiber, for example, has an index of just 51, compared to bran flakes' index of 74.

Therefore, you shouldn't assume that a food is good for you just because it's high in fiber. That's too simplistic. Study the glycemic index carefully, and learn to choose starchy foods that won't spike your insulin levels.

As a rule, it's easy to spot highly refined starches. You usually don't find them in your grocery store's produce section or in the whole-food bins; you find them on the shelves in boxes, mixes, and cans. Sometimes they've been precooked. They often boast of convenience: "Ready in 2 minutes!" More often than not, they're white: white bread, white rice, white crackers, pancake mix, rice cakes, potato chips, etc. The best way to avoid them is to buy *real* food—food that actually *looks* like food: potatoes instead of potato buds; fresh corn instead of corn chips; onions instead of frozen onion rings; bulk popcorn instead of caramel corn; raw nuts instead of beer nuts, etc.

It's also critically important to limit sugar. As we've noted, there are two foodstuffs that are most likely to derail your starch blocker diet: fat and sugar. If you can successfully control your intake of these two foodstuffs and are careful about neutralizing starch calories, you're almost certain to lose fat. But limiting sugar won't be easy. The average American diet is almost 25% pure sugar. So to succeed, you can't be "average" anymore.

Some strategists, it seems, start thinking of starch blockers as *carb* blockers, but that's a big mistake. Carbs include both starch *and* sugar, and there's no such thing as a sugar blocker. For several years, a substance called gymnema sylvestre was marketed as a sugar blocker, but it was never proven to be effective, and is no longer readily available. Similarly, there is also a product that's referred to as a fat blocker, called chitosan, but there's no compelling scientific evidence that it works.

It's unfortunate that there is no effective sugar blocker, because sugar is a national obsession in America. Consumption of it has almost tripled since the mid-1950s, amounting to an average intake of about 150 pounds per person annually in America—almost half a pound per day. Furthermore, refined sugar did not even exist until about 1,500 years ago—which was approximately 900,000 years after the human digestive tract was fully engineered by evolution. Without a doubt, the human body was not constructed by evolution in a manner that is compatible with high sugar intake. Like highly refined starchy foods, sugar throws the pancreas into overdrive, forcing it to pump out high levels of insulin, which layer on the body fat.

One major reason people now eat so much sugar is that huge quantities of it are "hidden" in processed foods. For example, catsup, mayonnaise, crackers, salad dressings, tomato soup, and barbecue sauce are often loaded with sugar, even though we usually don't think of them as sweet foods. To avoid hidden sugar, read labels carefully and remember that manufacturers often label sugar with an alias, such as sucrose, maltose, lactose, galactose, fructose, or high-fructose corn syrup. Look for "ose" at the end of an ingredient—it means sugar.

Fructose, or fruit sugar, has the best glycemic index at 23, and honey is next best, at 58. Because fructose has a relatively benign glycemic index, fruit is an acceptable component of the starch blocker diet. Some anticarb advocates regard fruit as little more than organic candy, but that perspective is irrational. The sugar in fruit is offset by its low glycemic index, the presence of fiber and amylopectin, and by the fact that fruit is often eaten raw.

Furthermore, many fruits are high in acid content, and acids appear to significantly reduce the glycemic impact of sugar, because acidic foods slow down digestion. It's been clinically noted that when a salad dressing with two tablespoons of vinegar was included with meals, it lowered the blood sugar response to the meals by 30%. Lemon juice was also shown to strongly delay delivery of food from the stomach to the small intestine. Therefore, including some vinegar or lemon juice in a meal that's high in sugar is probably wise.

Millions of people try to avoid sugar by using artificial sweeteners, but this seemingly smart strategy can backfire, especially for people with overly sensitive carbohydrate metabolisms. Artificial sweeteners such as aspartame (Equal) and saccharin have no calories, but several researchers assert that they still appear to trigger insulin overproduction in some people. The sweet *taste* of sugar substitutes apparently stimulates pancreatic production of insulin in sensitive people. However, when this insulin is produced, it has no dietary sugar to send into the body's cells. Therefore, it sends in the only sugar that's available: the sugar that's already circulating in the blood. This, of course, lowers blood sugar and can produce the uncomfortable symptoms of hypoglycemia: hunger, weakness, and irritability.

If people are already insulin resistant, this process can be even more harmful. In these people, millions of metabolically active cells, such as muscle cells, reject the blood sugar, and a disproportionate amount of it goes into the relatively more accommodating fat cells. Thus, among your cells, the fat get fatter.

There is also evidence that just the taste of sweetness, even in a calorie-free substance, evokes the extra endorphin output that typically occurs when people eat sugar. This can create the desire to eat even more artificially sweetened foods, or to eat other sweets.

Another potential weight-creating problem with aspartame, the most popular artificial sweetener, is that one of its primary ingredients is phenylalanine, an amino acid that is a nutritional precursor to the stimulating neurotransmitters dopamine and norepinephrine. Overproduction of these neurotransmitters can create a moderate high, akin to a "sugar rush," that can reinforce the desire for more foods with aspartame, or for more foods with the "real thing": sugar.

These factors help explain why artificial sweeteners haven't been shown by research to create or reinforce fat loss. In fact, in some studies, people drinking high amounts of diet soft drinks failed to lose weight or gained weight, while other people who were not using artificial sweeteners *lost* weight.

Therefore, there's a good chance that the various artificial sweeteners and diet soft drinks that you're now consuming may be working against you, instead of for you. The next time you drink a diet soda, pay careful attention to how you feel. If you get a temporary lift followed by a rebound feeling of hunger or discomfort, you should probably try to stay away from artificial sweeteners. If you do avoid both artificial and natural sweeteners, you'll probably miss them at first, and then will likely become increasingly indifferent to them. Right now, if you have a big "sweet tooth" problem, it may feel as if you could *never* become indifferent to sweets. But you can. It happens to thousands of people every day.

The starch blocker will help by significantly improving the function of your carbohydrate metabolism, giving you the extra edge you need in your battle against sugar.

Artificial sweeteners, though, aren't the only types of food that can cause you to experience adverse reactions and derail your starch blocker strategy. A number of extremely common foods can do this—anything from wheat to milk to eggs. In fact, the more common a food is, the more likely it is to be a culprit.

THE COMMON CULPRITS: REACTIVE FOODS

The most common foods in the American diet cause widespread food reactions and create terrible problems. These food reactions are a common cause of weight gain, and they greatly magnify the problems caused by a poor carbohydrate metabolism. Often, food reactions and excess carb consumption go hand in hand.

There are two kinds of food reactions: food allergies and food sensitivities. Some doctors call all food reactions "allergies," because that's a common term everyone understands. It's more accurate to refer to them by different names, though, because even though they have relatively similar symptoms, they have somewhat different biological causes.

Food allergies are very uncommon, and usually cause dramatic symptoms, such as hives or wheezing. Food sensitivities, though, are *quite* common, and can sometimes be more subtle. It's quite possible that you have at least one food sensitivity. The symptoms may be mild, but they may also be very noticeable. Many people have these symptoms quite often, but just take them for granted and don't link them to their cause. The most common symptoms of food sensitivities are heartburn, gas, bloating, swollen feet and hands, breast swelling, nasal congestion, fatigue, muscle weakness, joint pain, a puffiness in the face, a double chin, and watery eyes. These symptoms tend to occur soon after eating, but they can last from meal to meal, and be present almost perpetually.

The symptoms of food sensitivities occur when you eat something that your body cannot completely digest. When digestion is incomplete, large food macromolecules enter your bloodstream. The body perceives these macromolecules as foreign invaders, similar to viruses or bacteria. Your immune system then kicks into action with an inflammatory response and tries to flush the invaders out of your system, causing the uncomfortable symptoms.

As you know, starch blockers also create incomplete digestion, which results in the presence of large starch molecules. These large starch molecules, however, are eliminated before they can enter the bloodstream. The only people who are reactive to starch blockers are those who have an allergy to kidney beans, which is quite uncommon.

Several factors are responsible for the incomplete digestion that triggers food reactions. One cause is eating too narrow a range of foods. The average person gets about 75% of his or her calories from just ten different foods! When this happens, it can exhaust the body's ability to digest one or more of those particular foods.

Another cause is that we often just don't have enough of the enzymes that we need in order to completely break down foods. To help with this, you may wish to buy digestive enzymes at a health food store.

Genetic heritage also plays a role. For example, the ancestors of most African Americans consumed far less milk than the ancestors of most Caucasians, so now African Americans are ten times more likely than Caucasians to be reactive to milk. By the same token, millions of people are reactive to wheat, because it's only been around for about one one-hundredth of human history.

The other reason food reactions are so widespread now is that we eat too many artificial foods and too many highly refined foods.

When food reactions hit, they cause not only an immune response, but also a disruption of mood chemicals. They trigger release of a quick burst of insulin, which causes blood sugar to spike, then drop. There's also a spike-and-drop in endorphins, and in the contentment neurotransmitter serotonin. These chemical reactions are extremely similar to those that occur when too many carbohydrates are eaten.

There's only one quick, temporary fix for this disruption: Eat *more* of the reactive food, or eat a lot of carbs. Both of these quick fixes will mask the symptoms, but will cause them to quickly return, even more strongly.

This ugly partnership between reactive foods and high carb

intake overcomes the best intentions of many people. It doesn't just cause hunger, but a genuine craving, almost like the craving a drug addict experiences.

Therefore, to fully succeed on the strategy, you've got to stop eating the foods you're reactive to. It's not very hard to figure out which ones are the culprits. Here's a clue: In all probability, you're reactive to one of the six usual suspects.

THE SIX USUAL SUSPECTS

1. Dairy products

2. Wheat

3. Corn

4. Soy

5. Eggs

6. Peanuts

The other most common reactive foods are shrimp and other shellfish, chocolate, yeast, tomatoes, aspartame, gluten (in wheat, rye, barley, and oats), citrus fruits, monosodium glutamate, and additives such as dyes and sulfites.

The easiest way to find out what you're sensitive to is to contact one of several laboratories that specialize in food reactions. These labs will tell you how to send them a blood sample, drawn by your own doctor. For access to the labs, see Appendix A.

These tests can be moderately expensive, though, so many people try to figure out their reactive foods themselves. The best way is by doing an elimination diet, in which you stop eating your suspected reactive foods and see if this makes any difference in how you feel. If you do this, you should restrict all suspected reactive foods at once, for about a week, and then add them back to your diet one at a time, every few days. This can be difficult, but extremely revealing.

If you do find you feel better when you avoid certain foods, we strongly recommend that you continue to avoid them. Food reactions can destabilize your starch blocker diet, because they're so similar to the reactions you get from eating too many carbs.

If you find that you are reactive to wheat, you may feel cheated: "Finally I can eat all the wheat I want using the starch blocker strategy—but I'm *allergic* to it!"

This is a bitter irony, no doubt about it. But there are many alternatives to wheat products. Rice bread, for example, is quite good. Similarly, there are dozens of alternatives to milk products, many of which you will grow to love.

Even if these restrictions are hard, they'll be worth it. They will make your strategy all the more powerful and easier to maintain.

SUPPLEMENTING YOUR STARCH BLOCKER DIET

People who claim they get 100% of the nutrients they need from their diet alone must eat a lot of sardines, kale, anchovies, wheat germ, brussels sprouts, brewer's yeast, and bone meal. The *real* American diet, in the real world, just doesn't include the omnipresent, wide array of micronutrients the body needs to achieve optimal health, and to provide the energy it takes to stay slim and fit. Therefore, use of food supplements is important.

You don't need to take dozens of pills a day. However, you do need to take a multivitamin and mineral tablet at least once a day. By this, we don't mean taking the well-advertised, sugary little types of vitamins that contain only enough nutrients to keep people from contracting vitamin deficiency diseases, such as scurvy. We mean potent, powerful supplements purchased at a health food store or at a high-quality nutrition section of a grocery store. Scan the list of nutrients in the pills carefully. If they provide only a moderate percentage of the recommended daily allowance, they won't be strong enough to power you through another day of losing weight and feeling great.

In addition, you should take a B-complex vitamin in the 50-mg. to 100-mg. range. Even good multivitamins rarely contain enough of the B-complex to ensure the energy and mood stability that B-vitamins provide.

Other adjuncts to this basic level of supplementation could include:

- **Coenzyme Q-10**—a terrific energy builder that heightens the function of your cells' "power plants," the mitochondria: 100 mg. daily.
- **DHEA**—a hormonal supplement that's been shown to increase muscle mass and reduce body fat. DHEA, however, can exacerbate existing prostate problems, so it's not for everyone: 25 mg. daily.
- **Essential fatty acids**—which help the body burn fat and produce energy: 500 mg. twice daily.
- **Chromium**—a mineral that significantly aids the stabilization of blood sugar: 200 mcg. three times daily.

These special nutrients will make you feel better, increase your energy, and help you lose fat. Take advantage of their power.

SUCCESS IS NEVER EASY

When you write a book that charts new scientific territory and advocates a new strategy against an old problem, as Cameron Stauth and I are doing, you always try to imagine what the criticism of it will be.

In this case, it's easy. Cynics, as well as some well-meaning skeptics, will say: "*You're making it too easy!* This is salvation in a bottle! A pill for every problem! The only thing fat people need is *discipline,* not a miracle pill."

Having seen the starch blocker diet, can you honestly agree with this? We're insisting that you be almost ascetically moderate in your consumption of fat and sugar, if you plan to succeed. Right now, if you are an "average" American, fat and sugar comprise about 50% of your diet. We're asking you to whittle that to 27% of your diet (even *before* caloric neutralization of starch). Will that be *easy*? Probably not.

Thankfully, though, you've finally got a real ally in your fight against fat: the starch blocker. The starch blocker will allow you to compensate for the avoidance of fat and sugar with extra consumption of starchy foods. By *shifting* calories—away from sugar and fat to starch (and then neutralizing the starch calories)—you'll have a proven, scientifically sound method of eating normal amounts of normal foods, and still losing fat.

If your carbohydrate metabolism is currently dysfunctional, as it is for most overweight people, you'll finally have the same advantages enjoyed by people with a good carb metabolism. You'll be able to eat a plate of spaghetti or a sub sandwich without going into the danger zone of insulin overproduction. You won't get hungry a couple of hours later and start craving more carbs ("That spaghetti was great, but what good is spaghetti without some spumoni?").

You will, for once, be on a level playing field.

How well you succeed on that field is up to you. If you just use starch blockers as a way to cram down even more calories, you'll lose your fight against fat.

You'll probably also lose your fight if you don't join the battle with your entire being: your body, your mind, and your spirit.

You might have to change. Try a new lifestyle.

Are you ready to change the way you live?

The next chapter will help.

FIVE

STEP TWO: TAKING EMOTIONAL CONTROL

How Starch Blockers Give You Power over Food

'm starting to hate myself," my mother said.

"Hate yourself?"

"It's the weight. No matter what I do, I can't get rid of it."

"Mom, you're seventy-eight. It doesn't matter."

"It matters."

She was right, of course. Moms usually are.

She began to tell me about all the diets she'd been trying. The list went on and on.

"Your dad's been doing them with me," she said. "He's got twenty-five pounds to lose, if he's got an ounce. It's getting him down, too."

"I know something you should try."

"My son, the doctor."

I started telling her about starch blockers, but she rolled her eyes—the same way she had 30 years earlier, when I'd first mentioned the then-unknown science of acupuncture.

But my mother is a pragmatic person, a real problem solver, and after listening carefully she asked, "You're sure they'll help? I just feel so . . . out of control. We're both trying so hard."

"They'll help."

They did help. Within 12 weeks, my mother lost 10 pounds, and my father, who's 80 but exercises every day, lost about 20.

Even before they lost fat, though, they both regained their precious sense of having power over their own bodies.

According to the conventional wisdom of weight management, people first lose weight, and then regain their sense of physical efficacy, or control over their bodies. That's conventional thinking because that's the way it usually happens. But that's the hard way to regain power over your body.

The easier way—the smarter way—is to first level the playing field of metabolic function by taking starch blockers, and allowing this scientific breakthrough to prime the pump, so to speak, of personal power.

When starch blockers renew the biochemical efficiency of the body's carbohydrate metabolism, they give people a huge psychological boost. People feel in power again.

Furthermore, with regular use of starch blockers, mood impediments such as low serotonin levels, unstable blood sugar, and disrupted endorphin production are generally vanquished. This paves the way for an improved psychological outlook and for improved health behaviors, such as increased exercise and decreased eating.

Thus, in the strategy, physical success spurs psychological success.

Once strategists achieve their newfound sense of *psychological* well-being, it then reinforces their *physical* well-being, creating an upward spiral of strength and control.

Other types of successful weight loss diets can also help people to feel in control, but among all the dietary approaches that we now know of, the starch blocker strategy is uniquely effective at helping people gain power over their emotions, because of its singular effects upon mood chemistry.

Starch blockers improve mood chemistry primarily by correcting and stabilizing the levels of three of your body's most powerful forces: (1) the neurotransmitter serotonin, (2) blood sugar, and (3) the endorphins. When these mood-influencing forces are functioning smoothly, people are tremendously empowered in the fight against fat. They have the biochemical lift that they need in order to change their emotional and behavioral patterns. When they get this biochemical support, it often becomes relatively easy for them to lose fat. Often, for the first time, they enjoy the same buoyant mood chemistries that are more common among thin, energetic people.

TAKING CONTROL: THE THREE FORCES
THAT PUT MATTER OVER MIND

Force #1: Serotonin

The most significant advance in the field of psychiatry in the past fifty years was the introduction of medications that improve serotonin function. These drugs, such as Prozac and Paxil, stabilize levels of serotonin, the neurotransmitter that is the single most important chemical in the body for enabling people to feel contented and calm.

Millions of people, however, unknowingly wreak havoc upon their own serotonin systems because of the way they eat. Serotonin levels in the brain can plummet because of problems with carbohydrate metabolism.

One common problem is not getting enough carbohydrates, as sometimes happens to people who are on the more extreme low-carb diets. Carbs are necessary for carrying to the brain the nutritional building block that creates serotonin. This building block, or nutritional precursor, is tryptophan.

However, tryptophan, which is abundant in turkey, milk, and other high-protein foods, can't always enter the brain from the bloodstream because many other amino acids are competing with it. Here's how to make sure enough tryptophan gets in: *Eat at least a small amount of carbohydrate at each meal, accompanied by protein.* Try to avoid meals that are all starch or all protein.

Here's why this works. When you eat carbs—even if you neutralize about 75% of them with starch blockers—your body responds by secreting insulin. If you're also eating protein, insulin will move the amino acids in the protein into your cells. However, the amino acid tryptophan is a larger molecule than the other amino acids, and much of it tends to remain in the bloodstream. When abundant amounts remain in the blood, tryptophan has a big advantage in getting to the brain. In effect, it "overpowers" the other amino acids.

This serotonin-enhancing effect is a major reason why people feel contented after a balanced meal containing both carbs and protein.

Diets that are extremely low in carbs, though, often fail to produce this increase in serotonin. That's a major reason why people on some low-carb diets sometimes feel restless, irritable, and not content with the meals they've eaten.

However, you don't need to be on a low-carb diet to have a deficit of serotonin. In America, tens of millions of people have this problem, for a variety of reasons. Lack of serotonin often accounts for the carbohydrate craving that so many people commonly experience. It's not the starch in a plate of pancakes that they crave, but the sense of contentment and well-being that the starch triggers.

Some people have a genetic predisposition for carbohydrate craving. These people are born with a gene called DRD2 (dopamine receptor gene two). This is a common gene that is often inherited. It's known as a "thrifty gene," because it causes the body to hoard food energy, as if a famine were occurring. One reason, in fact, why so many people have it is because we're all descended from the *survivors* of innumerable famines. Many of the ancient people who *didn't* have the DRD2 gene undoubtedly died in famines, ending the lineage of their potential genetic descendants. For thousands of years, having this gene was the kiss of good luck, but too often in our current environment of abundance, it's the kiss of death.

If you have this gene, you will be more likely to secrete too much insulin when you eat carbs. Unfortunately, the more insulin you secrete, the hungrier you'll eventually get. The net result is that you will tend to crave carbs and to gain weight easily. You'll also be more prone to diabetes—the ultimate disease of impaired carbohydrate metabolism.

There's no point in trying to figure out if you have this gene. You can't do anything about it if you do have it, and you already know if you have the general traits this gene contributes to.

Furthermore, even people who don't have this gene can still develop these traits, just by eating too many carbohydrates over too many years.

Chronic overconsumption of carbs not only harms the carbohydrate metabolism, but it can also destabilize the serotonin systems of people who once had stable, high levels of serotonin. A repeated pattern of excess carb intake can affect the serotonin system in much the same way that recreational drugs can alter neurotransmitter systems.

For example, cocaine causes rapid release of the stimulating neurotransmitter dopamine, but when cocaine intoxication ends, dopamine is significantly depleted. Similarly, marijuana stimulates the function of the primary thought neurotransmitter, acetylcholine, but when marijuana intoxication ends, acetylcholine is depleted, leading to temporary loss of short-term memory. The same general pattern can occur when people overeat carbs: A massive amount of serotonin is released, which causes feelings of pleasure, but this is followed by a depletion of serotonin, with accompanying anxiety, depression, and food cravings.

As you can see, the brain functions best when it gets *a steady supply of serotonin—not too much at once, and not too little.* One of the best ways to achieve this is to not metabolize too many carbs at once, or too few carbs over the course of the day. You need a healthy, steady, *limited* intake of carbs. Starch blockers will help you accomplish this.

Achieving this steady, high level of serotonin is, unfortunately, harder for women than for men. The primary reason for this is that the female hormone estrogen tends to destabilize serotonin levels, while the male hormone testosterone generally stabilizes them. Particularly, serotonin levels become markedly lower when estrogen levels *fluctuate,* as they typically do during certain phases of the menstrual cycle. This largely accounts for the anxiety and depression often associated with premenstrual syndrome, or PMS.

This biochemical assault on the serotonin levels of females appears to have a widespread physical and emotional impact that goes far beyond uncomfortable PMS. It makes women more prone to a generalized variety of physiological dysfunctions. The first report of this generalized dysfunction syndrome appeared in Cameron Stauth's *The Pain Cure,* in which he noted that *low serotonin levels* are the common denominator in a number of maladies that had previously been considered unrelated—*all* of which have a far higher incidence among women than men. Among these conditions are clinical depression, which is 300% higher in women than men; chronic pain (300% higher in women); migraine headaches (1,000% higher); and irritable bowel syndrome (300% higher). All of these disorders have other causative elements, including psychological causes. However, there is absolutely no evidence that women are, in general, less psychologically stable than men. Furthermore, numerous studies have indicated that when serotonin levels were stabilized in women with these conditions, the conditions generally became far more benign and responsive to treatment, and frequently abated altogether with no adjunctive therapies.

Monthly hormonal fluctuation, with attendant serotonin deficits, is now widely believed to account for the food cravings that women commonly experience prior to menses. As a rule, these food cravings are centered on carbohydrates, because carbs provide a quick burst of serotonin production, as well as increases in endorphins and blood sugar.

Also, it's been noted that most *overweight* women generally prefer carbohydrates as their favorite type of food, while overweight men tend to prefer high-fat foods. This, again, is probably a result of biochemical forces that have nothing to do with aesthetic preferences for food tastes and textures.

It's long been known that women have a greater incidence of overweight and obesity than men. This, too, may be largely related to serotonin instability in women, accompanied by relatively more consumption of carbohydrates. For many years, it was assumed that weight management was essentially just a matter of willpower: pushing away from the table and getting up to exercise. This perspective now seems naive—even puritanically punitive. The playing field of weight management is not level. Women have more challenges than men.

The good news is: Starch blockers are 100% as effective for women as for men. They help level the field.

Force #2: Blood Sugar

The instinctual desire to produce serotonin is not the only thing that drives people to crave carbs. People are also driven by carbohydrates' unique abilities to produce other calming biochemical reactions.

The most obvious of these reactions, which you've probably experienced many times, is a rapid rise in blood sugar. This creates a neurological "carb rush" that can become as addictive to some people as the euphoria caused by recreational drugs.

When blood sugar, or glucose, rushes into the brain cells and muscle cells, it provides a huge mental and physical boost. Glucose is the only energy-releasing fuel that the brain and muscles receive, and when this fuel arrives in abundant quantities, the entire body, including the brain, responds positively.

The brain is even more sensitive to blood-sugar spikes than the body's other organs, because it uses more blood than any other organ—a full 25% of all the blood pumped by the heart. Therefore, when the brain gets a big, sudden blast of glucose, it "shifts into overdrive." Cognitive ability and mood soar.

However, blood sugar spikes are invariably followed by slumps, due to corresponding production of excess insulin. When this happens, the energy-producing "power plants" in brain cells, known as mitochondria, are hit hard. They don't have enough glucose to adequately perform complex mental tasks, store memories, or produce neurotransmitters. This causes mood impairment, irritability, lassitude, and inability to focus.

If brain cells are starved of glucose for more than just a few minutes, they begin to die. Over the course of your life, you've probably lost millions of brain cells because of depleted blood sugar. People who crash-diet are particularly vulnerable to this loss of brain cells.

Lack of glucose also has a terribly distressing impact on muscle tissues, including those that compose your major organs. When your muscles are starved of fuel, you feel weak, tired, lethargic, and shaky.

To compensate for lack of blood sugar, the body generally releases stimulating hormones, such as cortisol, which trigger the release of more insulin. This insulin then squeezes every available drop of glucose out of your blood for absorption into your cells. But these stimulating hormones, also known as stress hormones, generally make you feel even more shaky and irritable, as the last reserves of your blood sugar are exhausted.

When this occurs, it severely erodes willpower, and causes intense cravings for food.

The only way to overcome blood sugar spikes and slumps—and the food cravings they cause—is to stabilize levels of glucose so that there's never a time when cells run out of fuel. Starch blockers are uniquely effective at stabilizing glucose levels, by flattening the glycemic curve.

This stabilization results in a generally buoyant mood, elevated energy, good cognitive function, and physical strength and endurance. When these traits are present, people no longer need to "self-medicate" their irritability, depression, weakness, and lassitude with food—particularly with high intake of carbohydrates.

They have renewed power over food.

Force #3: Endorphins

The third major biochemical force that is triggered by excessive consumption of carbohydrates is release of a flood of endorphins. However, like spikes of serotonin and blood sugar, endorphin spikes are invariably followed by slumps.

The carb-endorphin connection was proven by researchers at McGill University. They monitored the carb intake of a strain of mice that have extremely low levels of endorphins, the body's natural, opiatelike painkiller. These low-endorphin mice, called C-57 mice, appeared to "self-medicate" their low-endorphin disorder by cramming down carbohydrates. They were carb junkies. They loved carbs and ate them compulsively. When they ate carbs, it didn't just bring their endorphin levels up to the normal range, it sent them rocketing off the charts. For these mice, sugar and refined starch were almost as potent as heroin—and were just as addictive. The C-57 mice would do almost anything to get carbs.

The C-57 mice were also very prone to addiction to alcohol. They became quite intoxicated very quickly compared to other mice, and preferred to remain intoxicated, even when alcohol began to destroy their health.

Yet another interesting aspect of this experiment was the inability of the C-57 mice to take control of their own environments. When researchers challenged C-57 mice and a control group of other mice with difficult or uncomfortable environments, the other mice scurried around looking for solutions, while the C-57 mice hunkered down helplessly in a passive posture.

So which came first for these mice—their behavior of helplessness or their biochemical dysfunction? That may sound like an unanswerable, chicken-or-egg question, but there is an apparent answer to it that comes from another, similar experiment.

This other experiment was a continuation of some of the most important psychological experiments ever conducted. The experiments were performed by Dr. Martin Seligman, who's been hailed by *Newsweek* as "The Freud of the 21st Century." Dr. Seligman's experiments provided the basis for his now-popular theory that depression and other mental problems often begin when people *learn* to feel helpless. "Learned helplessness," he believed, occurs when people experience too many no-win, double-bind situations. To test the theory, he placed one group of dogs in boxes from which there was no escape, and placed another group in boxes that did allow escape. Then both groups of dogs were subjected to mild electric shocks from the floors of the boxes. The dogs that could escape jumped out, but the ones that couldn't laid down and passively accepted the shocks. They had apparently learned to be helpless.

Then Seligman put *all* the dogs in boxes that allowed escape. Again, he shocked them. The dogs that had learned to escape jumped out, but the dogs that had learned helplessness stayed put, whining miserably, doing nothing.

Later on, other researchers added a twist to the experiment. They took a group of dogs that had learned to be helpless, but injected them with opiates that were chemically similar to their body's own endorphins. When they did this, the dogs quickly found a way to escape the shocks. The dogs, it appeared, had "unlearned" their learned helplessness.

The implications are profound! If the lessons from these experiments apply to humans—as the researchers believe they do—it indicates that when people are hobbled by dysfunctional contentment biochemistry, they are far more prone to feeling helpless, and to participate in their own self-destruction not only with passive behavior, but also with behaviors—like those of the "alcoholic," carb-addicted, C-57 mice—aimed at relieving their biochemical discontent. Among these self-destructive behaviors are eating too many carbohydrates and drinking too much alcohol. In humans, these behaviors would also presumably include using recreational drugs.

If this premise is true, there should be a link between alcohol addiction, drug addiction, and carbohydrate addiction. There is. Many studies have shown that a disproportionate number of people with poor carb metabolisms suffer from substance dependence. In my own practice, I have seen this link many times. In fact, it's typical for someone who is recovering from drug or alcohol addiction to overeat carbs. The carbs seem to offer a substitute high.

Similarly, people with dysfunctional carb metabolisms are also far more prone to addiction to caffeine and nicotine, which also temporarily confer contentment.

For many years, psychologists ascribed this pattern of generalized addictiveness to the psyche. They said people who were prone to addictions had "addictive personalities." It is far more accurate, we believe, to say that these people have addictive *biochemistries*.

This is a blessing! Why? Because biochemistry is easier to change than personality. Over the past twenty years, has your basic personality changed much? Probably not. You are who you are. But your biochemistry is almost certain to have changed. The combined assaults of stress, aging, and eating too many carbs have probably damaged the biochemistry of your carbohydrate metabolism. Sometimes you might feel like a "carb junkie" yourself, out of control of your eating habits.

If so, we have some good news.

HOW STARCH BLOCKERS HELP BREAK PHYSIOLOGICAL CARB ADDICTION

Starch blockers will markedly reduce mood swings and food cravings caused by dysfunctional carb metabolism. They will help stabilize your levels of serotonin, blood sugar, and endorphins. They will help pull you off the roller coaster of mood highs and lows that can destroy your sense of self-control. They can help change any feelings of learned helplessness that you may now be experiencing into an attitude of confident self-determination. That confident attitude was probably there all along, but for years it may have been buried beneath an avalanche of biochemical disturbance.

On a purely physical level, starch blockers will alter the way your body is accustomed to looking for fuel. Right now, if you're a heavy carb eater, here's the order in which fuels are used by your body.

THE BODY'S FUEL PREFERENCE—
BEFORE STARCH BLOCKERS

1. Dietary carbohydrates

2. Stored carbohydrates (glycogen)

3. Dietary fat

4. Dietary protein

5. **Body fat**

6. Body protein

That's how you've *trained* your body to act, by years of fueling it with quick-burning carbs.

Here's how this fuel hierarchy changes when you use starch blockers, along with a high-protein, moderate-fat diet.

THE BODY'S FUEL PREFERENCES—
AFTER STARCH BLOCKERS

1. Dietary protein

2. **Body fat**

3. Dietary fat

4. Stored carbohydrates (glycogen)

5. Dietary carbohydrates

6. Body protein

When carbohydrates are limited by starch calorie neutralization, it's not particularly hard for the body to train itself to use body fat as a primary source of fuel. Your body *likes* to burn body fat. It's a very efficient and accessible fuel. Unfortunately, though, you've probably trained your body *not* to convert body fat into energy, due to your steady intake of carbs. When carbs are readily available, your body will always go for them first, the same way a child will usually choose dessert over dinner.

Starch blockers, however, will retrain your body.

As they do, they will also enable you to retrain your mind.

Once you break your addiction to carbs—which may take a few days and be rather uncomfortable—you will no longer make the same mental associations with carb intake that you once did. You won't get the familiar blood sugar carb rush every time you eat a plate of pasta. You won't get a serotonin spike. Your endorphin levels won't rocket.

Maybe you'll miss these pleasures. People sometimes do. But like all artificial elevations of mood, these transient highs come with a big price—one you'll no longer have to pay. You won't pay the price of a rebound low—as serotonin, blood sugar, and endorphins sag back down, and then keep falling to distressingly low levels. Nor will you pay the price of guilt, as your temporary indulgence turns quickly into permanent fat.

Most gratifying of all, your mind will become free from the biochemical forces that may once have controlled it. You won't find yourself making elaborate rationalizations for why it's okay to do things you shouldn't, such as eating that extra plate of pancakes. Compulsion will be replaced by choice. When you are truly free to choose, you will probaby make wise choices. Self-destruction is almost never a free choice. It's practically always a compulsion.

As starch blockers allow you to break free of the biochemical compulsion to overeat carbohydrates, you will naturally begin to retrain your body.

As we mentioned, starch blockers retrain your body to prefer to burn body fat, instead of the easy fuel of carbohydrates. In effect, they get your body "hooked" on a new way of producing energy.

Once you start burning energy this way—from stored fat instead of from gobbling carbs—you'll feel different. There will be no more wild energy swings. No more mood swings. No more cravings. No more sluggishness. No more feeling out of control. No more guilt.

Best of all, no more of that terrible feeling with which you've probably become so familiar: *hunger.*

NO MORE HUNGER

Does it often seem to you as if the thin people you know never seem to get hungry? If so, it's not necessarily an illusion. In general, most thin people really *don't* get hungry in the way that you probably do. They usually have good appetites, they like food, and they look forward to eating. But they don't typically suffer the same urgent feelings before mealtime or snack time that are commonly experienced by many people with impaired carbohydrate metabolisms. Between meals, people with impaired carb metabolisms frequently feel all of the noxious symptoms caused by unstable levels of serotonin, blood sugar, and endorphins: weakness, shakiness, irritability, and anxiety. For them, hunger *hurts.* They feel as if they have hollow pits in their stomachs. Their hunger is not just a simple desire for food, but a biochemical *need-to-feed response.*

It's no coincidence that thin people generally don't experience the need-to-feed response. They often are thin precisely because they *don't* usually feel this way.

When people *do* feel like this, they *eat.* And they usually don't stop eating until the feelings go away.

This isn't weakness, and it's certainly not gluttony. It's as natural as putting a burned hand in cool water, or rubbing a fresh bruise.

With starch blockers, though, you can conquer the feelings that you now identify as hunger. You'll still have an appetite, and you'll still enjoy eating. However, you won't feel an urgent compulsion to eat, and you won't want to overeat.

Overeating only feels good when your carbohydrate metabolism is dysfunctional. When you're riding the roller coaster of physical and mental highs and lows that is caused by impaired carb metabolism, overeating during a meal or snack is one of the few times you really feel satisfied. When you take starch blockers, though, you will lose your chronic feeling of metabolic dissatisfaction. You'll begin to feel *uncomfortable* when you overeat. You'll feel stuffed—the same way thin people feel when they overeat.

One important reason you'll feel satisfied from a moderate intake of food is that you'll no longer suffer chronic, nagging deficits of serotonin, blood sugar, and endorphins. There is more than this, though, to feeling satisfied from hunger.

You also feel a state of satisfaction from food, medically known as satiety, because of the actions of key hormones. Production of these hormones generally starts with simply having a full stomach. When your stomach and small intestine are full, they begin to stretch, and to activate nerve endings in their smooth muscle linings. These nerve endings are known as "stretch receptors." The stretch receptors are connected by nerve pathways to the brain. When the brain receives signals from the stretch receptors, it naturally shuts off the desire to eat.

There are also stretch receptors in your lungs, and you can feel the power they exert just by breathing. Take a relatively deep breath, and you'll notice that you have a natural desire to stop inhaling, even though there's still plenty of room left in your lungs for more air.

The stretch receptors in the stomach and small intestine are just as powerful as the stretch receptors in your lungs. When they're triggered, they almost always make you want to stop eating, as long as you aren't suffering from the metabolic dysfunction of low serotonin, blood sugar, and endorphins. In fact, there's a valid new approach to weight management called "volumetrics," which revolves around filling the stomach and small intestine with high-volume, low-calorie foods, such as fibrous vegetables, in order to achieve satiety.

One of the problems with conventional low-calorie diets is that they just don't provide enough volume of food to adequately trigger the stretch receptors. Similarly, some of the low-carb, high-fat diets are also relatively low in food volume. A lack of food volume can make people feel as if their stomachs are empty, even when sufficient calories are present.

In contrast, starch blockers allow for consumption of relatively large volumes of food, without the accompanying large numbers of calories. They even *increase* the volume of starchy foods somewhat by allowing starch to pass through the system in whole-molecule form.

When the signals from the stretch receptors reach the brain's hunger center (the hypothalamus), the brain orders the release of the hormonal satiety signals. The satiety signals consist of short-term, medium-term, and long-term hormones.

The short-term hormone is CCK (cholecystokinin), which tells you it's time to end your meal. At the same time CCK is released, the brain turns off the production of a hormone that contributes to hunger, called ghrelin.

The medium-term hormone that's released is called PYY3–36, which suppresses appetite and helps keep you from being hungry between meals.

The brain then orders the release of a hormone that helps kill hunger for several hours. This hormone, leptin, also increases the rate of your metabolism.

The medical profession has tried to control hunger by administering these hormones as drugs, but it hasn't really worked. It's often quite difficult to trick the brain into a feeling that isn't really natural.

The advantage of the starch blocker strategy is that it doesn't try to trick the brain. It works in strict accord with the body's own natural processes. It satisfies the body's normal desire for fullness in the stomach and small intestine, without adding unnecessary calories. It also satisfies the natural emotional desire to eat a pleasurable, fulfilling diet, thus helping control psychological hunger.

Neurobiologist Dennis Meiss, Ph.D., has studied the effects of starch blockers on hunger, and has been very impressed. He has stated, "According to the clinical studies that have been performed, starch blockers appear to consistently lessen the extent of the peaks and valleys of glucose and insulin response that are typically seen following the ingestion of relatively high amounts of starch. Those dramatic peaks and valleys lead to extreme variations in insulin, other hormones, blood sugar, endorphins, and neurotransmitters. They cause people to suffer elevated sensations of hunger.

"Starch blockers help end that hunger."

When you begin taking starch blockers, you won't be "hooked" on carbohydrates anymore.

You'll feel energized. Alert. Content. Strong.

You will, in essence, get hooked on a *new* feeling. It will be even more powerful than the old feeling you got from a carb rush. It will be the rush you get from optimal health—an exquisite feeling of vitality, power, and clarity.

We call this "getting hooked on thinness."

The starch blocker can make this experience possible.

But only you can make it happen.

CHANGING YOUR MIND

Starch blockers can help change the function of your brain, if you use them properly. But you'll probably need to change more than your brain to become fit and trim for the rest of your life. You may also need to change your mind.

The brain is just chemicals. The mind is much more. It is the sum total of who you are. It is the repository of all your experience, and all the lessons you've learned.

It may be time now for you to unlearn some of those old lessons. Not all of them are true.

Some are lessons you learned while your brain and body were under the influence of destructive forces, including the forces of carbohydrate addiction and serotonin depletion. These forces compelled your *brain* to tell your *mind* lies. Such as: "Eat more carbs—you *need* them." Or: "Don't stop eating—you're not full yet."

This was just the carbs talking. But you tried to make sense of it, as people always do. In doing so, you probably told *yourself* some lies. Such as: "The only way for me to get thin is to be hungry." Or: "If I can't control what I eat, I must be weak and lazy."

Overweight people commonly have beliefs that make fat loss quite difficult. Here are the worst of them.

TOP TEN LIES OVERWEIGHT PEOPLE TELL THEMSELVES

1. *If I lose weight, I'll be able to respect myself.*

No—it's the other way around. When you start respecting yourself, you'll take care of yourself, and stop doing the things that ruin your life, including overeating. Make a list of all the things you love about your-self. Make a list of all the things you hate about yourself. Then tear up the hate list—and put the love list where you'll see it every day. Accept yourself. It's the only way to be happy, and you'll never be thin until you're happy. Whether you're fat or thin, you still deserve your own respect. Don't make your weight more important than it really is. If you're a good, decent person, you have absolutely no reason not to respect yourself, and to demand respect from others.

2.   *If I lose weight, it will change my life.*

Reality: If you change your life, you will lose weight. Forget those commercials where somebody gets all teary-eyed about how their new thin body won them love and self-respect. In real life, it happens the other way around. First, you learn how to love and respect your-self; *then* you lose weight. In fact, one of the dirty little secrets of the diet industry is that a major reason people regain weight after a diet is that they had thought the weight loss would change their lives. When it didn't, they quit trying.

3.   *If I could just lose weight, I'll look almost perfect.*

The secret to perfection is knowing there's no such thing as per-fection. If you understand that secret, you'll have as perfect a life as possible. Perfectionism is just fear of failure, disguised as ambition. It's an illusion. A crippling illusion.

4.   *I can't lose weight without being hungry.*

In reality, you can't lose weight without being full. Satiety is the key to fat loss, not hunger. If you're hungry, sooner or later you'll eat. Everybody does. What's the *point* of being hungry every day? That's not living—it's suffering. Learn to live—not suffer. Learn to be full, by eating all that you need.

5.   *Food is love.*

That ended when your mother stopped feeding you. If you're still eating fattening comfort foods from Mom's home-cooking

menu, stop. That food is not your mother. Your *mother* is your
mother. If you need to get in touch with her, use the telephone.
Good advice, but easier said than done, right? Just about everybody
has comfort foods, don't they? The key is to *know* that you're com-
forting yourself, and know when to stop. If you get too much food
"comfort," you'll feel worse instead of better.

6. *Eating relieves stress.*

It did when it corrected the biochemical imbalances that once
plagued you—*before* you began using starch blockers. But now you
have a new carbohydrate metabolism, and more stability in your levels of serotonin, endorphins, and blood sugar. You won't get the
same carb rush anymore, so don't even try. To some extent, eating
will still relieve stress by providing pleasure, but there are dozens of
forms of pleasure that won't make you fat and regretful. You know
what you enjoy. Do it.

7. *It's not right to waste food.*

It's even worse to waste your health. If you feel guilty about not
cleaning your plate, ask yourself: "Will I be better off with this food
in my *body*, or in the garbage disposal?" Save your leftovers, even if
it's just two bites. Two bites might be enough to satisfy you later on
in the evening, when you feel like a snack. You won't need hot fudge
sundaes anymore. Your body won't require them, and you'll learn
not even to desire them. Whether your hunger is biological or psychological, it *must* be satisfied, and starch blockers will help you satisfy it.

8. *Fattening foods taste the best.*

Only if you're driven by biochemical forces, such as low serotonin. Once you correct your carbohydrate metabolism, you'll learn
to appreciate the exquisite subtleties and complexities of wholesome
foods. You won't be lured inexorably to the crude fare of fat, sugar,
and starch, which compose an average of 80% of the American diet.
You'll stop eating like a seven-year-old with a bag full of sourballs.

9. *I just don't have the willpower to be thin.*

You shouldn't need willpower to be thin. If you do, you're doing something wrong. In all probability, what you're doing wrong is living on the teetering edge of carbohydrate addiction. Break the addiction, and the tension you're accustomed to will cease. You won't have to fight your cravings all day long. They won't exist.

10. *I inherited my fat. There's nothing I can do.*

Until recently, that might have been true. There is a distinct heritability to impaired carbohydrate metabolism. But science has come to your aid, and now offers a solution. If you use it, you'll have the same chance to be thin that everyone else has.

THE NEW WORLD OF WEIGHT LOSS

Now you understand the psychological component of the starch blocker strategy. Different, isn't it? It was approximately 85% about what the strategy can do for you, and only 15% about what *you* need to do for you.

Of course, that 15% is vitally important. But it's nice to get some help with the mental element of weight loss, isn't it?

■

We're finished now with the first two of the three primary forces of the strategy: the dietary component and the mental component. It's time to learn about the third component.

It's exercise.

Without exercise, you probably won't succeed. Promoters of weight loss diets rarely mention that. But it's true.

Exercising can be tough, can't it? Want some good news, though? *Starch blockers can supercharge your exercise program.*

Read on, and find out how.

SIX

STEP THREE: BURNING BODY FAT WITH EXERCISE

How Starch Blockers
Supercharge Your
Physical Activity

I t's true: You'll probably never lose much weight until you begin to exercise regularly. That's just a fact of life, and any diet guru who says otherwise is lying. That's the bad news.

Here's the good news: Starch blockers will *amplify* your exercise. They'll turbocharge it. They will make exercise easier, and even more importantly, they will make exercise more *effective.*

Starch blockers make exercise more effective by encouraging your body to *rely upon body fat* as a primary source of fuel. When the body becomes accustomed to looking for energy from body fat, instead of carbohydrates, it becomes more efficient in its *use* of exercise.

For example, a woman who's not taking starch blockers might burn about two ounces of body fat from an hour of slow jogging, but a woman taking starch blockers might burn three or more ounces. Over the course of a month, when all physical activity is taken into account, this degree of difference can have a huge impact upon fat loss.

This accelerated fat loss among starch blocker strategists occurs for two essential reasons.

First: People who do not take starch blockers almost always have more stored carbohydrates in their systems than strategists do. These stored carbs, called glycogen, are found in the liver and the muscles. The body loves to use glycogen for energy, because it's so easy to burn. It's basically just predigested, pure calories, waiting to be used.

Athletes in endurance events often try to increase their levels of glycogen in order to have an easy source of fuel to burn throughout their events. They do this by eating high amounts of carbohydrates, a practice that's called carbo-loading.

This is a smart tactic for running a marathon, but it's the exact opposite of what a strategist wishes to achieve. Unfortunately, in our current carb-obsessed culture, tens of millions of people carbo-load every day—without running marathons. People who are trying to lose fat want to burn as *little* glycogen as possible, and proceed to body fat burning as quickly as possible.

The only realistic way to do this is to have a limited amount of glycogen in the system. Starch blockers are uniquely adept at helping people lower their glycogen levels, by blocking unnecessary dietary carbohydrates.

The second major reason why strategists achieve accelerated fat loss from exercise is that their bodies become *biochemically trained to rely upon body fat as a primary source of energy.* When people are not taking starch blockers and are eating typically high amounts of starch, their bodies are accustomed to burning carbohydrates first, and body fat significantly later. This hierarchy of fuel preference changes, though, when significant amounts of starch calories are neutralized. The body of a strategist is relatively less dependent upon glycogen for fuel, and also is less dependent upon dietary carbs, dietary proteins, and dietary fats. After two or more weeks of consistent starch blocker use, the body of a strategist becomes singularly capable of focusing upon body fat as fuel. Within individual cells, fat burning is heightened, as the cells' fuel-transforming mitochondria achieve maximum efficiency.

For many centuries, this degree of responsiveness to exercise was very much the norm. When our ancestors were physically active, as they were so much of the time, they saw the results almost immediately, much the same way, for example, that a teenager with a still-undamaged carb metabolism might respond quickly to exercise.

However, as America's carb binge has become entrenched as the dietary standard over the past fifty years, the efficiency of exercise among many people has declined. It's now common for people on high-carb diets to exercise strenuously on a regular basis, but still be overweight. Much of the time, even when they exercise, they burn only glycogen and dietary calories (especially carbs), rather than body fat.

If you now respond poorly to exercise, you may have often felt frustrated when you've seen people at the gym who regularly do less work than you, but still look better. Perhaps you told yourself, "They're just lucky; they have a fast metabolism." Or, "They're younger—that's their advantage." In reality, though, their biggest advantage is probably a healthy carbohydrate metabolism. That's the kind of "luck" you can create by neutralizing starch calories.

Your natural responsiveness to exercise can usually be restored in as little as two to three weeks, with robust starch calorie neutralization.

However, because this process usually takes several weeks, we do not believe it is necessarily wise for people to begin to exercise during their first couple of weeks on the strategy. Exercise during this period won't do any harm, but it will not have as much positive effect as exercise done after the starch blocker has had time to elevate body fat burning in the hierarchy of fuel preference.

Therefore, exercise done a little too early in the strategy can sometimes be rather demoralizing. It can feel the same way it has for many years: You huff and puff, and barely lose an ounce.

Another good reason to hold off on exercise at first is that it will allow you to be certain that the starch blocker, by itself, is making a critical difference. Finding out for sure that you're finally getting some real help is always good for your morale.

In addition to helping make fat loss through exercise more biologically efficient, the strategy also makes exercise easier by ridding the body of the excess pounds it must carry during exercise. Exercise can be extremely difficult, even intimidating, for people who are 40 or more pounds overweight. It's like trying to exercise with a 40-pound pack on your back.

Finally, starch blockers make it easier to summon the *energy* to exercise. When people suffer from the conditions of impaired carbohydrate metabolism—such as hypoglycemia, hyperglycemia, Syndrome X, and diabetes—their glycemic highs and lows often drain them of the energy they need to exercise consistently. It's long been presumed that these people merely lacked willpower, but that judgmental perspective is flawed. For virtually everyone, willpower *starts* with energy.

Therefore, as you can see, starch blockers can, in effect, kick-start your exercise program. Then, once you're exercising regularly, here's what happens.

THE METABOLIC EFFECTS OF EXERCISE

1. **Exercise oxidizes calories.** It burns them faster than any other physiological action. The easy-to-remember equation on exercise and fat loss is: One hour of exercise each day burns one pound of fat each week. Over just four months, one hour of exercise per day creates 20 pounds of fat loss.

2. **Exercise reduces insulin levels.** It increases insulin sensitivity (the ability of cells to respond to insulin). This decreases the need for excessive insulin output. In addition, exercise burns body fat, and the less fat you have, the less insulin you produce. When there's less insulin in your system, your body is more prone to *burn* fat, instead of *store* it. Even when people don't lose weight, exercise still reduces their vulnerability to diabetes.

3. **Exercise increases muscle mass, which boosts calorie burning.** Muscle tissue burns fat approximately 10% to 20% more efficiently than any other body tissue, including body fat. This occurs even when the muscles aren't in active use! Because men generally have greater muscle mass than women, they have an advantage in caloric burning.

4. **Exercise stimulates fat-burning hormones.** One hormone is testosterone, the primary male hormone that is also present, in smaller amounts, in women. Testosterone builds muscle mass and increases energy and feelings of well-being in both men and women. Exercise also increases output of the stimulating hormones thyroxin and norepinephrine, which increase metabolic rate. In addition, exercise enhances the production of energizing

neurotransmitters, including dopamine. When all of these chemicals are released in a concerted symphony of metabolic enhancement, they rev up the metabolism by approximately 5% to 15% for about four hours. This increase in metabolic rate, over a period of months or years, accounts for vast amounts of caloric oxidation.

For spurring fat loss, those are the four most significant actions of exercise. However, exercise also has other critically important benefits, many of which have an indirect impact on fat loss. Here they are.

- **Exercise decreases appetite.**
  Conventional wisdom says that a good workout increases hunger, but science says it doesn't. The hormones and neurotransmitters associated with exercise all have a stimulating effect on the body and help control hunger in much the same way that stimulating dietary chemicals do, such as the caffeine in coffee. To contribute to hunger, exercise must be prolonged for several hours, thoroughly depleting glycogen, as well as most accessible body fat storage areas.

- **Exercise improves mood.**
  This can be vitally important for weight management, because depression and anxiety are the two most frequent causes of emotional overeating. Many studies demonstrate that regular, moderate exercise is generally as effective against depression as antidepressant medication. In one recent Duke University study, for example, 60% of people recovered from clinical depression by exercising only half an hour a day, three times a week, for four months. One reason for this antidepressive effect is the increased production of endorphins, which are boosted by 500% during vigorous exercise. In addition, exercise enhances production of stimulating catecholamine neurotransmitters, such as norepinephrine and dopamine. Exercise also has a profound impact upon cognitive function, or intellectual ability, due to its effects upon neurotransmitters and neuronal circulation. In *Brain Longevity,* Cameron Stauth and Dr. D. S.

Khalsa demonstrated that exercise is one of the most important factors for achieving optimal cognitive function and helping prevent Alzheimer's disease.

- **Exercise improves general health.**
  Everybody knows exercise helps prevent cardiovascular disease, the number-one killer in America. What many people don't know is that it also helps prevent the minor illnesses that account for most incidences of missed work and missed workouts. In one study, people who exercised missed about 20% fewer workdays than those who didn't. Other studies show that exercise reduces the risk of cancer of the reproductive organs by 250%, the risk of breast cancer by 200%, and the risk of colon cancer by 67%. It also significantly reduces chronic pain. Obviously, not all of these benefits are directly related to weight management. But they're certainly all related to health, and as we've mentioned, when optimal health is achieved, fat loss will tend to occur naturally, as an almost unavoidable consequence.

WHAT TO DO

To achieve the maximum benefit from exercise, try to do one hour of exercise every day. To many people, this sounds excessive, but it's not. It's a mere fraction of what mankind has been doing throughout our existence. For millennia, our ancestors were at least moderately physically active five to ten hours each day! We are programmed by evolution to require generous amounts of physical activity.

Further evidence that an hour a day is necessary comes from the U.S. government. The federal government has long been very conservative about the amount of exercise it recommends, but the 2002 federal guidelines on weight management recommended at least one hour per day—an increase of 100% over the federal guidelines released as recently as 1996.

Your one hour each day should consist primarily of moderately vigorous exercise. This is generally defined as exercise that increases resting heart rate by approximately 50%. For example, if your heart beats 80 times per minute while you're sitting, it should beat half again as fast—or 120 beats per minute—while you're exercising. If it is beating less than that, you will probably not deplete your glycogen during the exercise period, and will therefore not burn body fat.

In addition, exercise must be engaged in for at least 25 to 30 minutes at a time. Even among strategists doing moderately vigorous exercise, it will take at least this long to burn through stored glycogen and to begin oxidizing fat. For people who are not neutralizing starch calories, it will take even longer—up to 40 to 45 minutes.

Exercise *must* be moderately vigorous in intensity, but it may also be more strenuous. One of the modern myths of exercise is that fat can be burned *only* with moderately vigorous exercise, rather than strenuous exercise. In fact, strenuous exercise burns more calories than moderate exercise—it just burns them less efficiently in relation to the amount of work you're doing. For the most part, the harder you exercise, the more you will benefit.

It is quite possible, though, to exercise too much. Here are the warning signs of excess exercise.

- Prolonged fatigue, even after a day of rest.
- Presence of minor injuries.
- Muscle aches that won't go away.
- Increased resting heart rate.
- Loss of appetite.
- Mood disturbance, including depression and anxiety. (Too much exercise is as disconcerting to mood chemistry as too little.)

Most people are not ready to do a solid hour of exercise when they begin the strategy. It's typical, in fact, for people to be completely sedentary when they first begin various weight management programs. Obviously, their sedentary habits are typically part of the problem.

If you are not accustomed to exercise, a reasonable way to start is to just walk around the block. The next day, you should walk around it twice. By the end of the week, you should be walking around it three or four times, or about a mile.

Every week, the distance and speed should increase slightly. The key is to keep achieving steady increases. Each new level of activity tends to heighten the body's propensity for fat burning.

After a few months of regular exercise, most healthy people are quite capable of performing an uninterrupted hour of exercise. People who are significantly overweight will almost always perform their exercises more slowly than people who weigh less, but will still burn off even more calories than thinner people, simply because they're carrying extra weight with each movement. Therefore, overweight people benefit more from exercise than thin people, even though their objective performance levels are lower.

As soon as you feel ready, it's important for you to ratchet your exercise up to the huff-and-puff level. To achieve all its widespread metabolic benefits, exercise must be somewhat strenuous. If you're not breathing much harder than normal and not breaking a sweat, it's very possible you aren't pushing yourself hard enough. Don't expect exercise to always be easy. It takes effort. Good things usually do.

Some people find it's easier and more pleasant to alternate traditional aerobic exercise, such as jogging, with strength-building exercise. This is a good approach.

Conventional wisdom says that fat loss can only be achieved with aerobic exercise, which creates more oxygen use than strength-building, or anaerobic exercise. This perspective is flawed. One reason it's not true is because strength-building exercise builds muscle, and increased muscle mass contributes significantly to enhanced caloric burning.

Furthermore, the distinction between aerobic exercise and strength-building exercise is often rather contrived. It's almost impossible to perform a strength-building exercise, such as lifting weights, without experiencing an increase in respiration and heart rate, the two primary characteristics of aerobic exercise. Similarly, it's virtually impossible to do an aerobic exercise without moving one's own body weight, which is why aerobic exercises build muscle, similar to strength-building exercises. Thus, each form of exercise will help you do the other.

Therefore, you should just focus on staying active, instead of worrying about what activity to do.

Activity, of course, does not include the minutes you may spend waiting around to catch your breath after a strength-building exercise. To lose weight, you don't *want* to catch your breath. You want to keep moving. One of the most popular new exercise routines, in fact, combines using light weights *during* aerobic exercises. This approach is very effective.

One activity that won't achieve its intended effect, though, is focusing fat-loss exercise on a specific part of the body, such as the buttocks or abdomen. Even though TV commercials constantly imply that this is possible, there is no such thing as "spot reducing." Doing abdominal "crunches" will cause no more weight to be lost from your abdomen than it will from your buttocks or arms. The body simply doesn't oxidize fat in relation to the muscle groups that are being used.

Even so, it's quite possible to *tone* the muscles in specific regions, such as the buttocks, abdomen, hips, thighs, or arms. This generally improves the appearance of the area that is focused upon.

You may notice, though, that the weight from your abdomen might oxidize more quickly than the weight that's stored in your hips, thighs, and buttocks. Adipose tissue, or fat, in the hips, thighs, and buttocks tends to have higher concentrations of resistant fat, or "quiet fat," which is not as metabolically active as fat in the abdomen. In the abdomen, the triglycerides that compose fat are constantly being broken down and rebuilt, mostly to provide fuel. Lower-body fat, however, processes insulin even less efficiently than abdominal fat, and is therefore harder to break down.

Unfortunately, many women tend to store fat in these resistant areas. This is one of the special challenges that females face. For them, losing fat is even harder than it is for men.

THE CHALLENGES WOMEN FACE

Women generally carry more body fat than men. From an evolutionary survival standpoint, this was an advantage, because women have always needed fat in order to be fertile and to withstand the energy demands of pregnancy and breast-feeding. Breast-feeding, for example, requires an extra 500 to 1,000 calories per day, and pregnancy requires at least 10 to 12 extra pounds of body fat to ensure fetal health.

Body fat increases the production of estrogen, which is vital for fertility. Estrogen, though, causes even *more* fat to be stored. This commonly creates a recurring cycle of estrogen/fat/estrogen/fat, making weight loss quite difficult for some women.

If a woman's body fat percentage drops from the average of about 30% or 32% to below 20%, it has a markedly negative effect upon her fertility. If it drops to 12% to 15%, as it often does among female athletes, it can impair fertility and may cause total cessation of menstruation.

Even when females are first born, they have about 10% to 15% more fat than males. During puberty, their body fat increases by an average of about 50% as their estrogen levels rise. In contrast, when boys go through puberty, their increased testosterone allows them to build more muscle and to burn fat approximately 10% to 20% more efficiently than women.

Thus, by age 20, the average body fat ratio of women is about 20% to 25%, compared to 12% to 19% among men. By age 55, the average body fat percentage among women is 30% to 35%, compared to 23% to 28% among men.

Primarily because of these hormonal factors, approximately 25% more women are overweight than men.

When impaired carbohydrate metabolism combines with this natural hormonal propensity for women to gain weight, it can create a veritable "perfect storm" of fat storage. Willpower alone is rarely sufficient to tame this storm of adipose accumulation. The most willpower can do is to give someone enough strength to go on a very low-calorie diet, and even this difficult effort pays dubious dividends. When confronted with a very low-calorie diet, the body naturally increases fat storage even more, as if a famine were occurring.

Currently, the most effective way for women to defeat these powerful biological forces is to oppose them with an equally powerful biological force: the activity of the starch blocker, which neutralizes calories, helps repair carbohydrate metabolism, and helps oxidize the excess body fat that creates even more estrogen, and more fat.

COMBINING ALL THREE STEPS: CALORIC REDISTRIBUTION, TAKING EMOTIONAL CONTROL, AND EXERCISE

The exercise element of the strategy is tremendously important. To fully succeed on the strategy, though, you need to do more than just exercise vigorously. You need to actively implement all three steps of the strategy into your life. Let's quickly review them:

Step One: Caloric Redistribution. You can, with a moderate amount of effort, lose one-half to one pound of fat per week by shifting calories to the starchy foods component of your diet, and then neutralizing starch calories.

To achieve this degree of fat loss, you must eat prudently, limiting your intake of fat and sugar. Prudent eating is indispensable for a full, vibrant life, because how you eat reflects your whole approach to living. If you chronically overeat, there's something wrong with your basic approach to life, and you'll eventually pay the price of excess—in your weight and in your life. And forget junk food—that garbage is for people who will *always* be fat. Furthermore, if you think that you can eat starchy foods in gross excess, and then neutralize their calories, you probably won't be able to lose weight and keep it off. Excess always finds a way to ruin even the best-laid plans.

Step Two: Taking Emotional Control over Food. Starch blockers will prime the pump of your power over food by boosting your mood chemistry and helping to end your food cravings. This will give you the emotional strength you need to deal with food in the same general way that thin people do. Thin people don't live to eat—they eat to live. You can achieve this attitude, too, if you use starch blockers to remove the biochemical mood impediments that undermine willpower.

Step Three: Exercising. You can lose a pound a week solely from exercising one hour each day. We strongly recommend that you stick with this vigorous exercise regimen *even after you reach your goal weight*. If you do, you will feel better, look better, and be far healthier.

Exercise, as we've shown, affects far more than just body fat. It optimizes overall health, and compared to your general health, being somewhat overweight is *trivial*. (And by *health,* we don't mean merely "absence of disease." Health is *energy, power, zest . . . happiness.*) Get healthy, and thin will follow.

If you just can't, or won't, exercise this much, don't beat yourself up over it. Guilt is counterproductive. It's just another form of self-indulgence. Instead, do as much as you can. Fifteen minutes a day is *vastly* better than nothing, and half an hour is far better than fifteen minutes. Don't fall into the all-or-nothing trap. That's the kind of compulsive thinking that gets people into trouble with their health habits.

These are the three steps of the strategy. They can change your life.

Starch blockers can make this change easier.

If you're ready to change, keep reading, and we'll tell you the exact type of diet that will make this change possible.

PART THREE

GETTING STARTED

SEVEN

AN OFFICE VISIT

What You Need to Know
to Start the Strategy

It's time for you to start the strategy.

Imagine you're coming in to a clinic to find out how to begin. Here are the questions you'd probably ask. These are the typical, nuts-and-bolts issues that patients most often bring up as they prepare to set out on this revolutionary approach to weight management.

Q: Can I use starch blockers over a long period of time?

A: You can use them indefinitely, the same way you might use vitamin A to keep your eyes strong, or glucosamine to keep your joints healthy. People have taken starch blockers for years at a time with no ill effects, and there's no reason to expect that problems will arise in the future. After you reach your goal weight, though, you may wish to reduce your use of starch blockers, because you'll no longer be trying to lose weight. Often, people who reach their goal weights use starch blockers only once per day, at their largest meal of the day. This reduced use allows them to consume relatively more calories than they would be able to without taking starch blockers, thus making their mealtimes more pleasant and satisfying.

Q: How many starch blockers should I take?

A: The recommended dosage is two 500-mg tablets with each meal. That may be somewhat more than you need, but because there are no significant side effects, and because starch blockers are inexpensive, some people take even larger dosages than this, just to be absolutely sure they're blocking as many starch calories as possible. Nonetheless, taking more than three or four at even a very high-starch meal is probably a waste of money. If you do take an excessive dosage, though, there will be no negative side effects, according to current safety studies.

Q: Do I take them with all meals, or just starchy meals?

A: They only work against starch, but most meals contain at least a small amount of starch, even if it's not obvious. For example, almost all vegetables contain starch, and so do most fruits.

Q: If I take more than the recommended dosage, will I lose more weight?

A: No, you'll only be able to block the starch calories that are present at any one meal or snack and, for most starchy meals, two tablets will work as well as twenty-two.

Q: When do I take them?

A: Ideally, just before you eat. If you forget to take them prior to a meal, though, it's better to take them after you've already begun to eat than not to take them at all. When you do take them late, however, they're not as effective.

Q: Will it help to skip meals, or to fast, while I'm on the strategy?

A: No—it's counterproductive. We recommend eating regular meals. Eating regularly will stop your body from going into the starvation mode of caloric hoarding. It will also keep you from being hungry. Just be sure that you eat wholesome, low-fat, low-sugar meals and snacks.

Q: Isn't getting hungry a sign that you're losing weight?

A: No, it's just a sign that you're suffering. And if you suffer too long, you'll probably start eating more than you should. Being hungry doesn't make people thin. Being full does.

Q: Can exercise help me lose body fat?

A: Yes—especially on the strategy. The strategy prevents excess storage of carbohydrates and therefore encourages the body to burn body fat instead of stored carbs. You should be able to burn one pound of body fat per week from exercise alone. That would require an hour a day of moderate exercise.

Q: Do I have to count calories?

A: Not as carefully as you do on denial-oriented diets. Most people normally eat about 25% to 35% of their diets as starch, so they can expect to lose weight without making major dietary changes, as long as they don't overdo the fat and sugar. Working out a precise plan, though, is also quite easy. To figure out your own individualized weight management plan, see the next chapter.

Q: Even as a child I was overweight. Can starch blockers help me overcome my genetic tendency to gain weight easily?

A: They can. Part of your genetic problem is probably an impaired carb metabolism, as it is for most overweight people. The strategy will help correct it. It will train your body, possibly for the first time, to prefer to burn stored fat, instead of dietary carbohydrates and stored carbohydrates.

Q: How is this different from other diets?

A: It's more than a diet. It's a programmatic strategy consisting of three steps: (1) caloric redistribution, (2) taking emotional control, and (3) exercising, all done in conjunction with taking starch blockers. Starch blockers neutralize redistributed starch calories, make emotional control over food easier to achieve, and supercharge exercise.

Q: Will I have to use starch blockers for the rest of my life?

A: It won't hurt you in any way if you do, because they don't have significant side effects. However, your metabolism will probably respond to starch blockers by becoming more efficient, enabling you to use starch blockers much less frequently, particularly after you reach your goal weight. After an extended period of time, you might not need them at all.

Q: How will I know if I don't need them anymore?

A: If you become happy with your weight, and happy with the diet you're eating, you won't need them. This is not an uncommon occurrence. It's more common, however, for people to reach a weight they like, but still wish to continue to neutralize starch calories in order to be able to eat somewhat more indulgently, without gaining weight.

Q: How do I determine my goal weight?

A: You can start by figuring out your body fat percentage, according to the formula in Chapter Eight. When you compare your body fat percentage to that of other people, using the charts that accompany the formula, you'll get a good idea of how much fat you should lose. Even so, there is no mathematical assessment that will be as accurate as your own good judgment. You are the only person who really knows exactly how you want to look and feel. If you achieve a sense of well-being, you've reached your goal—no matter what you weigh.

Q: I've lost weight with a conventional low-carb diet. Can I combine starch blockers with that diet?

A: Yes. Starch blockers tend to work well with virtually all of the existing low-carb diets. They make them easier to follow, because you get to add starchy foods without adding all the extra starch calories.

Q: Do starch blockers block the other type of carbohydrate—sugar?

A: No, they have no effect on any food other than starch. There are products that claim to be sugar blockers and fat blockers, but there's no compelling scientific evidence that they're effective.

Q: If my weight hits a plateau, what should I do?

A: It's likely that you will hit plateaus occasionally and will stop losing weight for a week or more. If this persists for more than
about three weeks, you should adjust your ratio of calories
metabolized versus calories burned. You'll have to eat less, exercise more, or neutralize more starch calories. Remember, the
thinner you become, the fewer calories your body needs.

Q: If I use starch blockers with stimulant diet products, will I lose
weight faster?

A: We don't recommend this at all. Stimulants are almost never
effective for long-term weight management, and they have far
too many negative side effects. Stick with a natural approach,
and don't rush your weight loss. If you rush it, you'll regain
weight much more easily.

Q: It's *important* for me to lose weight as quickly as possible. Is
there any safe way at all to do this?

A: No. If you lose more than two to three pounds per week, you'll
hurt your body more than you'll help it. You'll trigger the starvation effect of caloric hoarding, making it extremely difficult to
keep weight from returning. You'll also burn muscle tissue
instead of fat, and when you regain weight, it probably won't be
lost muscle that you'll regain, but fat.

Q: Doesn't everyone want to lose weight quickly?

A: Only if their diets are making them miserable. The strategy will
have the opposite effect. You'll feel better on it. You'll actually be less
hungry than usual, with more energy and more mood stability.

Q: Do I need a prescription for starch blockers?

A: No, they're an over-the-counter, nonprescription supplement.
They're natural, nonstimulating, organic, nonallergenic for most
people, and contain no herbs that have powerful, druglike effects.

Q: Where can I get them?

A: They're available at most health food stores and at many pharmacies, discount stores, and grocery stores. Look for them in the diet section.

Q: Are some brands better than others?

A: At this point, we don't know about any cheap, knockoff versions, such as ones that are just ground-up kidney beans. However, it's almost inevitable that these will eventually creep into the marketplace, possibly via less regulated venues, such as the Internet. To protect yourself from these brands—which have not been proven effective by clinical studies—buy only brands containing Phaseolamin 2250 (also called Phase 2), which is the current most popular formula. This designation will be listed on the label. This is the standardized formula that has been widely clinically tested. To the best of our knowledge, no other formulas, at the time of publication of this book, have been clinically tested for weight loss in humans, with results reported in a scientific journal.

Q: Can starch blockers be taken by children? And what about women who are pregnant or breast-feeding?

A: Thus far, none of the studies on starch blockers have involved children, or women who are pregnant or nursing. Therefore, we do not feel comfortable recommending this. However, if a woman who is pregnant or breast-feeding wishes to discuss using starch blockers with her own physician, that doctor may feel it is acceptable, due to the general nontoxicity of starch blockers. Even so, pregnancy and breast-feeding are typically inappropriate times for any attempt at weight loss. Any significant degree of caloric reduction at this time could result in harm to both the woman and her child.

Similarly, it may be that some overweight children might benefit from starch blockers, but since this has never been studied, we do not advocate it. Parents may, however, wish to discuss the matter with their own pediatricians or family physicians.

Furthermore, while it's true that childhood obesity is a serious health problem, it's also true that childhood is a time of growth and development, which can be irreparably harmed if caloric needs are not met.

Q: Could starch blockers be abused by people with eating disorders?

A: In theory they could, although there are no reported cases of this. Because starch blockers neutralize starch calories, people could possibly binge on high-starch foods and then neutralize the calories, just as they could binge on low-calorie or calorie-free foods, such as diet sodas or nonfat potato chips. However, most people with eating disorders prefer to have empty stomachs, instead of full stomachs, so they might not be attracted by the strategy of caloric redistribution and neutralization.

Q: Don't starch blockers make losing weight too easy? Whatever happened to discipline and willpower?

A: Starch blockers make fat loss easier, but it's still a challenge. You've still got to control fat and sugar intake, and you still have to exercise. Starch blockers mostly just make the effort of weight management more fair—they help the bodies of people with impaired carbohydrate metabolisms to function more like the bodies of people with healthy carb metabolisms. Starch blockers level the playing field— but your success will still depend upon your own efforts.

Q: My family doctor is curious about starch blockers. How can she learn more about the scientific details?

A: She can review the studies in Appendix C, or she can read synopses of some of the safety and weight loss studies at www.starchstopper.com.

Q: What are the worst side effects that could occur?

A: The worst that have occurred in studies are minor bloating and gas, which have gone away after 24 hours, as people's bodies adjusted. Even minor reactions were rare, though.

Q: Can starch blockers be taken with prescription drugs without causing problems?

A: They have no known interactions with any prescription drugs.

Q: I've heard that some starch gets digested in the mouth, even before you swallow it. Will starch blockers stop this?

A: Some starch blockers are chewable, and they will inhibit starch digestion in the mouth. One chewable brand is Starch Away, a Phase 2–containing product, made by Leiner Health Products.

Q: I have diabetes. Can I count on starch blockers to keep my blood sugar stable?

A: Because diabetes can have deadly consequences, complete reliance upon starch blockers would be very unwise for people with this disease. For example, what if you ate more starch than you thought you had, or maybe took your starch blocker a little bit too late in the meal? For most people, these mistakes would be inconsequential. For someone with diabetes, they could be very problematic. Therefore, if you have diabetes, you should wait for more testing to be done, and for a protocol to be established. In the meantime, you still might benefit from starch blockers and might be able to enjoy a more varied diet containing more starch (if you neutralize the starch calories). But do not stop testing your blood sugar levels and do not alter your medical use of insulin without specific, explicit orders from your doctor.

Q: Are special foods that have been redesigned to be low in carbs, such as those commonly eaten by diabetics, compatible with the starch blocker diet?

A: Yes, they can be very helpful. Many people, including diabetics, add variety and flavor to their diets by eating food items such as cookies or cake in which high-carb grains and sugars have been replaced by substitutes such as soy and fructose. (Appendix A has more information on this.)

Q: Were starch blockers banned by the FDA in the 1980s?

A: No, but the FDA did order companies to stop claiming that they caused weight loss, because not enough clinical studies had been done. Now these studies have been done, using the one brand that is the most popular formulation of starch blockers (Phaseolamin 2250, or Phase 2), and weight loss claims can be made for products that contain this formulation.

Q: I've heard you can eat junk food on this diet, and still lose weight. True, or not true?

A: True, but you'll still be eating junk—just junk that's not quite as fattening. For example, if you eat full-fat potato chips on the strategy, you'll neutralize about half their calories. But the calories you'll absorb will be almost pure fat. Why do that? You might as well go eat a can of lard.

Q: Since beer is made from grains, such as barley, hops, and wheat, will starch blockers neutralize the calories in it?

A: No, the fermentation process changes the starch calories to a form of sugar. Starch blockers won't block any form of alcohol.

EIGHT

YOUR OWN DESIGNER STARCH BLOCKER DIET

Choose the Foods That Fit Your Needs

The rest of this book is nothing but action. From here on, we show you how to actively bring the strategy's power into your life.

In this chapter, we start by showing you how to figure out approximately how much body fat you now have. This will give you a close approximation of how much you should lose.

Then we tell you how to lose it. We give you a great formula for determining *exactly how much* to eat. You won't find a formula like this in any other diet book.

The rest of the chapter will help you decide *what* to eat. We have unique lists that you won't find anywhere else, such as one that delineates the exact number of starch calories in a wide variety of common foods.

In the next chapter, we show you how to design the menu plans that will get you to your goal weight. You'll love looking at our sample menus. You've never before seen so much food on any other weight loss menu.

In the last chapter, we offer more than 100 recipes that are especially tailored to the strategy. The recipes have a very special feature. They tell you exactly how many starch calories are in each dish, and how many are neutralized by the starch blocker. They're delicious recipes, many of which came from one of America's most outstanding chefs, Philippe Boulot.

From this point on, *you* are the driving force in this book. With the information we offer, you can create your own, individualized starch blocker diet, and integrate it into your lifestyle.

This will be one of the great adventures of your life.

HOW MUCH FAT SHOULD I LOSE?

It depends on how much you *want* to lose. People have different goals. Some people want to look like movie stars. Good for them— there's nothing wrong with having lofty goals. Other people have no interest in the realm of perfection, but simply want to be fit and trim. That's a great goal. It's attainable, practical, and is superb for general health. Others just want to stop being fat. *Good for them!* That's an excellent goal, worthy of serious effort. Anybody who can achieve this goal deserves admiration.

Determining your goal, though, takes a little preparation. It's hard to know where you want to go until you know where you are. Following is a formula that will tell you where you are on the relative scale of body fat. After you complete this formula, you'll know approximately how many pounds of fat are on your body, and what percentage of your entire weight that fat comprises. You'll then be able to compare yourself to other people, using a chart we provide.

Some people are surprised to learn they're carrying so much body fat. If you find that you're fatter than you thought, don't be discouraged. On the strategy, you'll be more in control of your weight than ever before, and you will have the power to *change your life.*

Determining your percentage of body fat, and comparing it to that of other people, will help you determine your goal weight. But it will not be the sole determinant. Your final goal is *up to you.*

Every goal is worth reaching.

You can start the process of reaching your goal today.

Estimate Your Percentage of Body Fat

A. Multiply your waist measurement   _____
    (at the level of your navel) by 4.15.   (Answer A)

B. From this figure, if you are a male,   _____
    subtract 98.42. If you are a female,   (Answer B)
    subtract 76.76.

C. Multiply your body weight   _____
    by .082.   (Answer C)

D. Subtract Answer C from   _____
    Answer B.   (Answer B)

                                   − _____
                                        (Answer C)

Your pounds of body fat.   (equals) =   _____
                                                    (Answer D)

E. Divide your pounds of body fat
    (Answer D) by your weight. Your
    percentage is the first two numbers
    after the decimal point.

    Your pounds of body fat: _____
                                       (Answer D)

                               ÷ _____=_____
                                  (your weight) **Your Body Fat
                                                   percentage**

Example

A man weighs 175 pounds and has a 34-inch waist.

A. 34 (inch waist) times 4.15 = 141.1.

$$\frac{141.10}{\text{(Answer A)}}$$

B. 141.1 minus 98.42 = 42.68.

$$\frac{42.68}{\text{(Answer B)}}$$

C. 175 (pounds of body weight) times .082 = 14.35.

$$\frac{14.35}{\text{(Answer C)}}$$

D. 42.68 (B) minus 14.35 (C) = 28.33.

$$\frac{28.33}{\text{Pounds of Body Fat}}$$

E. 28.33 (pounds of body fat) divided by 175 (pounds of body weight) equals 0.1618, or 16% body fat.

$$\frac{.1618 \text{ or } 16\%}{\text{Body Fat percentage}}$$

Now that you know your body fat percentage, see how it stacks up against that of other people.

Body Fat Rating Scale

Males

Age	Excellent	Good	Fair	Poor
19–24	10.80%	14.90%	19.00%	23.30%
25–29	12.80%	16.50%	20.30%	24.40%
30–34	14.50%	18.00%	21.50%	25.20%
35–39	16.10%	19.40%	22.60%	26.10%
40–44	17.50%	20.50%	23.60%	26.90%
45–49	18.60%	21.50%	24.50%	27.60%
50–54	19.80%	22.70%	25.60%	28.70%
55–59	20.20%	23.20%	26.20%	29.30%
60+	20/30%	23.50%	26.70%	29.80%

Females

Age	Excellent	Good	Fair	Poor
19–24	18.90%	22.10%	25.00%	29.60%
25–29	18.90%	22.00%	25.40%	29.80%
30–34	19.70%	22.70%	26.40%	30.50%
35–39	21.00%	24.00%	27.70%	31.50%
40–44	22.60%	25.60%	29.30%	32.80%
45–49	24.30%	27.30%	30.90%	34.10%
50–54	26.60%	29.70%	33.10%	36.20%
55–59	27.40%	30.70%	34.00%	37.30%
60+	27.60%	31.00%	34.40%	38.00%

Information extrapolated from various sources. See chapter notes in Appendix B.

HOW MUCH TO EAT

Now it's time for you to determine exactly *how much* you should eat and *what* you should eat.

To figure out how much to eat, you'll need to fill in some of the simple formulas that we've provided. You'll love doing them. They're very precise, and very revealing.

Once you know how much to eat, you can devise your own eating plan by choosing among the multitude of food lists we provide in this chapter. The food lists tell you which foods work best for people on the strategy. In fact, we've even given them grades of A through F, to help you rank their compatibility with the strategy. We also tell you exactly how many starch calories are in practically all common, starchy foods and how many *total* calories these foods contain.

Equipped with this information, you will find it easy to create your own "designer" starch blocker diet, tailored to your own biological needs, tastes, and food preferences.

Then, in the next two chapters, we'll give you suggestions for combining these foods into complete menu plans, and we'll give you a comprehensive selection of delicious recipes.

Over the next year, as you integrate the strategy into your lifestyle, you'll probably refer to the information in these last few chapters many times. It's extremely useful.

Let's get started!

■

Let's get down to the nuts and bolts of exactly how much you should eat.

You will find that the following formula that determines your daily caloric needs is quite simple. If you can add, subtract, multiply, and divide, you can do it. It's much easier, of course, to do it with a calculator, and we recommend that you use one.

Don't be put off by the length of it. Most of the reason why it's rather lengthy is that it's all stated so simply. Making things easy takes up space.

When you're done, you'll know something very valuable: the exact number of calories per day that your own body needs to meet the demands of your own particular job activities, after-work activities, and exercise activities.

As you may have noticed if you've read a number of other weight management books, no other book contains a formula that tells you exactly how much to eat, based on your own individualized needs. The primary problem with this lack of direction is that it leads to many people eating too little or too much. Both are equally harmful. If you eat even slightly too much, you'll gradually gain weight and give up in frustration. If you don't eat enough, you'll destabilize your metabolism by triggering your body's caloric hoarding response, and end up gaining weight instead of losing it. For permanent weight loss, slow, steady decline is the way to go.

As you work through the following material, keep in mind that this is the amount of calories you need to *remain at the weight you are now.* To lose weight, you will need to either cut calories or increase your current activity and exercise levels.

Calories are simply a measure of the amount of energy food provides. The more calories you eat, the more energy you are giving your body. This energy must be used, or it will be stored as fat. If you are trying to maintain your current weight, you should metabolize the same amount of calories that you expend each day. If you are trying to lose weight, you should metabolize fewer calories than you expend.

Daily Caloric Needs

There are four basic components that make up your body's energy expenditure. They are: **basal metabolic rate, job activity level, after-work activity level,** and **exercise level.** By adding these four basic components, you will be able to find how many calories your body needs each day. Complete each step below in order to arrive at your personal level of energy expenditure.

1. **Basal Metabolic Rate (BMR).**
    This is the amount of calories your body needs to maintain the basic "housekeeping" of survival. This includes such things as heartbeat, breathing, maintaining your body temperature, and manufac-

turing hormones. It is the amount of calories you need just for sitting still or lying down. Surprisingly, this accounts for *60% to 70% of all calories expended.* To find your basal metabolic rate, follow these equations. Note that they differ for men and women.

For adult males:

A. Multiply your body weight by 10 (for example, a 175-pound man = 1,750).

B. Then double your body weight (175 × 2 = 350).

C. Now add the totals from A and B (1,750 + 350 = 2,100 calories).

D. For every decade you are over age 20, multiply the total calories from C by .02. Then subtract this number from C (if the man in our example is 40 years old: 2,100 calories × .04 = 84; 2,100–84 = 2,016 calories). If you're near a midpoint in a decade, such as near age 35, age 45, age 55, etc., multiply by .025, .035, .045, etc. This will give you your total basal metabolic rate.

Your BMR = _____ (male)

For adult females:

A. Multiply your body weight by 10 (for example, a 130-pound woman = 1,300).

B. Then add your body weight to this value (1,300 + 130 = 1,430 calories).

C. For every decade you are over age 20, multiply the total calories from B by .02. Then subtract this number from B (if the woman in our example is 40 years old: 1,430 calories × .04 = 57; 1,430–57 = 1,373 calories). If you're near a midpoint in a decade, such as near age 35, age 45, age 55, etc., multiply by .025, .035, .045, etc. This will give you your total basal metabolic rate.

Your BMR = _____ (female)

2. Job Activity Level: Which One Fits You?

A. *Sedentary Job:* This would include a desk job or any type of office work. Jobs that may be sedentary would include that of a student, an attorney, an accountant, a telemarketer, or a computer technician.

   Give yourself a 1.1 if you fit this category.

B. *Light Physically Active Job:* This would be a job that requires being on your feet at least half the day, such as that of a sales-clerk, a teacher, homemaker, cook, doctor, nurse, typist, beautician, or a factory worker who is seated but uses his or her hands while working.

   Give yourself a 1.2 if you fit this category.

C. *Moderately Active Job:* This type of job involves a moderate amount of brisk or challenging physical activity throughout the day. It would include the jobs of auto mechanic, plumber, carpenter, lawn and garden maintenance worker, mail carrier, or a factory worker who does frequent, light lifting.

   Give yourself a 1.3 if you fit this category.

D. *Very Active Job:* This type of job includes strenuous activity, such as that required in the fields of landscaping, farmwork, construction, logging, heavy warehouse work, or heavy factory work.

   Give yourself a 1.4 if you fit this category.

Note: If you fall somewhere at a midpoint between these four basic categories, you can adjust them accordingly by adding another modifying digit to your Job Activity Level score. For example, if you do somewhat more than what we describe as a Light Physically Active Job—but still don't reach the level of a Moderately Physically Active Job—you can add a modifying digit to your score of 1.2, such as: 1.21, 1.22, 1.23, 1.24, etc.

The job activity levels also apply to people who are retired, or who are otherwise not employed, but are still physically active.

   Your Job Activity Level: _____

3. **After-Work Activity Level**

   When you're done working for the day, which description fits you best? Do *not* include your daily workout or exercise routine in this; exercise is calculated in the next category.

   A. *Couch Potato:* You do as little as possible, other than to watch TV, read, or engage in other sedentary activities. Give yourself a score of 0.0.

   B. *Household Helper:* Somebody else does the housework and plays with the kids, but you try to help out as much as you can, and you stay moderately busy during much of the evening. Give yourself a score of 0.01.

   C. *Go-Getter:* You're on your feet all evening long, like it or not. You make dinner, do the dishes, tend to the kids, shop for groceries, mow the lawn, and do the housework. Give yourself a score of 0.02.

   Your After-Work Activity

   Level Score = _____

4. **Exercise Activity Level**

   Using the chart below, add all the calories you burn each day via exercise. Don't forget incidental exercise, such as walking somewhere for lunch or walking your dog. If you only do this exercise every other day, divide your score by 2. If you exercise less than that, adjust your score accordingly (for example, if you only exercise one day per week, divide your numerical calorie score by 7). As you'll note, the weights increase in 25-pound increments, and the calories increase in 50-pound increments. Therefore, for every pound of weight you are in excess of the closest listed weight, add two calories. (For example, if you weigh 101 pounds, instead of 100, and play baseball, give yourself a score of 219 instead of 217.)

Calories Burned by Exercise in One Hour
According to Body Weight

Weight	100 lbs	125 lbs	150 lbs	175 lbs	200 lbs	225 lbs	250 lbs	275 lbs	300 lbs
Activity									
Baseball/Softball	217	267	317	367	417	467	517	567	617
Basketball	450	500	550	600	650	700	750	800	850
Bowling	170	220	270	320	370	420	470	520	570
Chopping Wood	294	344	394	444	494	544	594	644	694
Cross-Country Skiing	500	550	600	650	700	750	800	850	900
Cycling 13 m.p.h.	560	610	660	710	760	810	860	910	960
Elliptical Trainer	805	855	905	955	1005	1055	1105	1155	1205
Fast Jogging	580	630	680	730	780	830	880	930	980
Football	430	480	530	580	630	680	730	780	830
Gardening	118	168	218	268	318	368	418	468	518
Golf	145	195	245	295	345	395	445	505	545
Heavy Aerobics	444	494	544	594	644	694	744	794	844
Heavy Calisthenics	444	494	544	594	644	694	744	794	844
Heavy Weight Training	512	562	612	662	712	762	815	862	912
Housecleaning	172	222	272	322	372	422	472	522	572
In-line Skating	500	550	600	650	700	750	800	850	900
Light Aerobics	104	154	204	254	304	354	404	454	504
Light Calisthenics	172	222	272	322	372	422	472	522	572
Light Weight Training	172	222	272	322	372	422	472	522	572
Medium Aerobics	240	290	340	390	440	490	540	590	640
Medium Jogging	512	562	612	662	712	762	815	862	912
Medium Weight Training	342	392	442	492	542	592	642	692	742
Rowing Machine	550	600	650	700	750	800	850	900	950
Sex	47	97	147	197	247	297	347	397	447
Slow Jogging	376	426	476	526	576	626	676	726	776
Swimming 2.5 m.p.h.	199	249	299	349	399	449	499	549	599
Walking 3.75 m.p.h.	199	249	299	349	399	449	499	549	599
Yoga	140	190	240	290	340	390	440	490	540

From Hatfield, F. C., *Fitness: The Complete Guide*. International Sports Sciences Association, 2002. Used by permission.

Your Exercise Activity Level = _____
                                                              Expressed as calories

Now jot down all four of your Activity Levels.

1. **Basal Metabolic Rate** =   _____

2. **Job Activity Level** =   _____

3. **After-Work Activity Level** =   _____

4. **Exercise Activity Level** =   _____

Here's how to figure your daily caloric needs. Use the workspace below.

1. Add your **Job Activity Level** and **After-Work Activity Level.**

2. Take the *total* from step one, and *multiply* it by your **Basal Metabolic Rate (BMR).**

3. *Add* to this your **Exercise Activity Level.**

Here's your workspace:

Step 1.

_____ + _____ = _____
Job Activity Level   After-Work Activity Level   Total

Step 2.

_____ × _____ = _____
Total from Step 1   Basal Metabolic Rate (BMR)   Total

Step 3.

_____ = _____ (same number as Exercise
Exercise Activity   Total   Activity Level)

Step 4

_____ + _____ = _____

Total from Step 2   Total from Step 3   **Your Daily
Caloric
Needs to
Maintain
Your Body
Weight**

An equation for this would be:

(Job Activity Level + After-Work Activity Level) × Basal
Metabolic Rate + Exercise Level = Daily Caloric Needs to
Maintain Body Weight.

For example:

1. Sarah weighs 140 pounds and is 46 years old, so her BMR is
   1,471 calories.

2. Her Job Activity Level is a Light Physically Active Job, so this
   means she gets a 1.2 rating.

3. Her After-Work Activity Level is household helper, so she gets an
   0.1 rating.

4. Her Exercise Activity Level is 350 (or 350 calories burned daily).
   So to calculate her total daily caloric needs, all Sarah needs to do
   is put these numbers into the equation: (1.2 + 0.1) × 1,471 +
   350 = Sarah's daily caloric needs. It would look like this: (1.3 ×
   1,471) + 350 = 2,262 calories needed per day to maintain
   Sarah's body weight.

QUICK AND DIRTY CALORIC NEEDS EQUATION

(For the Mathematically Challenged)

You can also get a good estimate of your daily caloric requirements using one of these simple formulas. It's not as accurate, but it's usually relatively close.

For sedentary people: Weight × 14 = estimated calories needed per day.

For moderately active people: Weight × 17 = estimated calories needed per day.

For active people: Weight × 20 = estimated calories needed per day.

This is a good, simple way to figure your changing caloric needs on a weekly basis as your weight drops.

Information extrapolated from various sources. See chapter notes, Appendix B.

LOSING WEIGHT

Now you know how many calories you need to *maintain* your body weight and keep from gaining. But you want to *lose weight*, right? Figuring out how much less you need to eat is easy.

As you probably remember, 3,500 calories equals one pound of body fat. Eat an extra 3,500 calories, and you'll gain about a pound. Burn 3,500 calories with extra exercise, and you'll lose about a pound. Or *neutralize* 3,500 starch calories from your normal diet, and you'll lose about a pound.

To lose one pound per week, you'll need to burn, neutralize, or not eat 3,500 extra calories each week—or 500 each day.

WHAT TO EAT

We believe that one-size-fits-all diets are generally ludicrous. Different people need far different amounts of food, based upon their individual metabolic needs, and different people have vastly varying tastes. Therefore, we think the smart way for you to have a good, prudent diet is for you to design it yourself. Ultimately, that's what virtually everyone does anyway, isn't it? When was the last time you faithfully followed a weight loss menu plan for more than about a week—if *that* long? Following diet plans is just too complicated and too restrictive, and it doesn't take your own desires and lifestyle into account.

There are four main factors to consider when designing your own starch blocker diet: (1) The speed with which foods enter the system and trigger insulin spikes. This is called the glycemic index. (2) The relative abilities of various foods to satisfy hunger. This is called the satiety index. (3) The number of starch calories in each food. (4) The total number of calories in each food.

Let's look at each of these four factors. After we do, you'll have a clear idea of which.

THE GLYCEMIC INDEX: FAST FOOD AND SLOW FOOD

As we mentioned earlier, there are stark differences in how quickly different foods enter the bloodstream and cause elevations in blood sugar and insulin levels. Some foods dash into the system; some stroll in at a leisurely pace. You should eat foods that enter slowly, because they will be least disruptive to your metabolism and most supportive of a stable mood and high level of energy.

The entry speed of foods is rated according to a glycemic index. In this index, all foods are rated in comparison to pure sucrose, or table sugar, which has an index of 100. Therefore, if a food has an index of 50, it enters the bloodstream half as quickly as table sugar, and is therefore healthier.

Because you'll be neutralizing about 75% of your starch calories, the glycemic index won't matter as much to you as it would to someone who metabolizes all of his or her starch calories. Even so, you'll still metabolize about 25% of the starch calories you eat, so you'll want them to creep into your bloodstream as slowly as possible.

Surprisingly, many starchy foods enter the system almost as quickly as sugar. Often, foods that seem as if they'd be good for you actually have higher glycemic indexes than seemingly unhealthy foods. For example, rice cakes have a glycemic index of 87, while frosted flakes have an index of 55.

Most foods made from rice, in fact, have high glycemic indexes. Rice cereals, such as Rice Chex™ and Puffed Rice™, have indexes in the 80s. Instant rice, and pasta that is made from rice, have indexes in the 90s. Brown rice is the only type of rice with a low index (59).

Most breakfast cereals also have high indexes. Besides the rice cereals, others with indexes in the 80s are cornflakes, Corn Chex®, Crispix®, Team™, and Grape-Nuts® Flakes. Most other cereals are in the 70s. The only cereals with good, low indexes are oatmeal (49) and All-Bran® (44).

Another category of food with a high, unhealthy glycemic index is bread (including crackers, pancakes, and waffles). For the most part, the glycemic indexes of breads are in the low- to mid-70s. This includes whole wheat bread, which has the same glycemic index as white bread (72). The only types of bread with moderate indexes are pumpernickel (49), whole rye (50), and pita (57).

Candy and other sweets also generally have very high glycemic indexes, in the range of 70 to 80. However, when candies or other sweets contain nuts, which slow down digestion, the index drops by about half. The index of a nut-filled Snickers® bar, for example, is 41.

Similarly, dessert-type foods that contain both sugar and starch have high indexes. Most types of cookies tend to be in the 70s, and cakes are generally around 55–65. The presence of oil or butter in cakes and cookies slows digestion somewhat, however, and keeps the index from being even higher.

Fruits, in general, have good, low indexes, though certain types are better than others. The highest are notably sweet fruits, such as dates (103), watermelon (72), cantaloupe (65), and raisins (64). Tropical fruits, such as bananas (62), pineapples (66), papayas (58), and mangoes (55), tend to have higher glycemic indexes than fruits from moderate climates, including apples (38), pears (36), plums (24), strawberries (32), peaches (42), apricots (30), and cherries (22). An exception to the rule that tropical fruits have higher indexes is grapefruit, which has an index of only 25, due to its relatively low sugar content.

The best glycemic index ratings belong to beans and vegetables, which are often high in fiber and protein. For example, soybeans have an index of 10, and kidney beans and red lentils have indexes of 27. Others with indexes in the range of 30 to 40 include lima beans, navy beans, split peas, chickpeas, and hominy. Vegetables, in general, have low glycemic indexes, and are therefore excellent as components of the starch blocker diet. Examples include yams (51), unpeeled white potatoes (63), sweet potatoes (54), sweet corn (55), beets (64), and carrots (49). Potatoes that are peeled, however, have notably higher glycemic indexes. Peeled mashed potatoes have an index of 86, and peeled, red-skinned, boiled potatoes have an index of 88.

Thus, in regard to glycemic index, these foods are most appropriate for the starch blocker diet in the following order, from best to worst:

GLYCEMIC INDEX RATINGS
(FROM BEST TO WORST)

1. Beans

2. Vegetables with peels intact

3. Peeled vegetables

4. Moderate-climate fruits

5. Nonrefined, bran cereals

6. Whole rye, pumpernickel, and pita breads

7. Wheat breads (including whole wheat and white), crackers, and pancake mixes

8. Sweets with nuts and fats added

9. Brown rice

10. Tropical fruits

11. Very sweet fruits (melons and raisins)

12. Refined breakfast cereals

13. Rice cereals

14. Rice pasta, rice cakes, and instant rice

15. Table sugar, or pure-sugar candies with no nuts or fat added

(Information extrapolated from various sources. See chapter notes, Appendix B.)

THE SATIETY INDEX: FOODS THAT FIGHT HUNGER

Some foods are more "filling" than others. The ability of various foods to satisfy hunger, or induce satiety, was recently quantified by a panel of European physicians. In the index they created, all foods were compared to ordinary white bread, which was assigned an index rating of 100. Therefore, for example, oranges, which have a satiety index rating of 202, are about twice as filling as white bread.

Until this index was devised, conventional wisdom held that high-sugar and high-fat foods were good for satiety. However, the doctors discovered, from interviews of patients who had recently eaten, that sugar and fat are not really very filling, despite all the calories they contain.

High-sugar foods temporarily calm hunger pangs by spiking blood sugar and insulin. However, this spike is invariably followed by a drop, which makes hunger even worse. Also, like high-fat foods, sweets usually don't have a lot of bulk, so the stomach and small intestine quickly feel empty and relay these sensations to the brain, where they're interpreted as hunger.

Cake, as an example of a sweet food, has a satiety index rating of only 65, indicating that it's significantly less satisfying than white bread. Doughnuts have a similarly low rating (65), as do many types of candy bars.

Foods are more filling when they're packed with fiber and protein.

Therefore, fruits, which are often just as sweet as cake, have a much better satiety rating than cake. In addition to oranges, satisfying fruits include apples, with a rating of 197, grapes (162), and bananas (118).

Many high-starch foods have good satiety ratings, especially if they are made from whole grains. Whole wheat pasta has a rating of 188, whole wheat bread has a rating of 157, and brown rice has a rating of 132. Even refined starchy foods are relatively capable of satisfying hunger. While rice has a rating of 138, white pasta has a rating of 119, and french fries have a rating of 116.

Some starchy breakfast cereals, when served with milk, are also good at satisfying hunger, especially if they're not refined. Oatmeal has the highest satiety rating of any cereal, at 209, and All-Bran® has a rating of 151. Cereals that are more refined get lower scores. Even so, cornflakes (118), Special K® (116), and Honeysmacks® (132), are still more filling than bread.

Starchy snack foods are also relatively filling. Popcorn is best at 157, and crackers are relatively close behind at 127. Nuts, which are high in fat but low in volume, do not score as favorably. Peanuts, for example, have a satiety index of 84.

High-protein foods are easily the most filling foods. Lentils have a satiety rating of 133 and baked beans score 168. Eggs have a 150 rating, and cheese has a 146 rating. Beef goes all the way to 176, and fish tops the list as the most satisfying food, with a satiety index of 225.

Here's a quick rundown of common food categories and foods, based on their ability to induce satiety, ranked from best to worst.

SATIETY INDEX
(FROM BEST TO WORST)

1. Fish

2. Oatmeal

3. Beef

4. Beans

5. Eggs

6. Popcorn

7. Cheese

8. Lentils

9. Brown rice

10. Crackers

11. Cookies

12. White pasta

13. Cornflakes

14. Bananas

15. French fries

16. Special K®

17. White bread

18. Ice cream

19. Peanuts

20. Candy bars

21. Doughnuts

22. Cake

(Information extrapolated from various sources. See chapter notes, Appendix B.)

The Starch Calorie Index

This chart, painstakingly compiled, is unique. You won't find it in any other books or among readily accessible sources.

For you, it's absolutely vital, because it's your only practical resource for determining the amount of starch in your food. Without it, you won't be able to participate in the strategy with precision and accuracy.

Bear in mind that these calories are for starch alone—not carbo-hydrates, which consist of starch plus sugar.

Using this guide, you can easily devise your own meal plans with exactitude and confidence.

STARCH CALORIE INDEX

BEANS (½ CUP COOKED, OR AS NOTED)

	starch calories	starch grams		starch calories	starch grams
anasazi beans	72	18	navy beans	88	22
azuki beans	72	18	pinto beans	80	20
black beans	72	18	refried beans	84	21
black-eyed peas	60	15	soybeans	24	6
chickpeas/garbanzo	84	21	split peas	72	18
great northerns	68	17	tempeh (3 oz)	40	10
kidney beans	72	18	tofu, firm (3 oz)	4	1
lentils, green	72	18	tofu, reduced fat (3 oz)	16	4
lentils, red	80	20	tofu, silken soft (3.5 oz)	10	2.5
lima beans	68	17	tofu, silken extra	10	2.5
mung beans	72	18	firm (3.5 oz)		

BREADS (1 SLICE EACH, OR AS NOTED)

	starch calories	starch grams		starch calories	starch grams
bagel, sprouted spelt	178	44.5	French bread	72	18
bagel, sprouted wheat	120	30	mochi, plain (1 piece)	96	24
bagel, white	148	37	mochi, sesame garlic	92	23
bagel, whole wheat	116	29	(1 piece)		
crackers, rye crisp-bread (1)	24	6	mochi, raisin-cinnamon (1 piece)	86	21.5
crackers, rye thin crisp (4)	24	6	naan ™	132	33
			pita, whole wheat	96	24
crackers, stoned wheat (2)	20	5	pita, white unenriched	128	32
			rice cake, no salt	56	14

BREADS (1 SLICE EACH, OR AS NOTED) *continued*

	starch calories	starch grams		starch calories	starch grams
rice cake, w/salt	56	14	tortilla, spelt	104	26
rye bread, typical	40	10	tortilla, sprouted wheat	56	14
rye sourdough bread	88	22	tortilla, whole wheat	80	20
tortilla, blue corn	88	22	white bread	44	11
tortilla, corn	116	29	whole wheat bread	100	25

FLOUR (¼ CUP)

	starch calories	starch grams		starch calories	starch grams
amaranth flour	76	19	rice (brown) flour	120	30
arrowroot flour	112	28	rice (white) flour	112	28
barley flour	76	19	rye flour	80	20
buckwheat flour	80	20	semolina flour	80	20
carob flour	92	23	soy flour	20	5
chickpea flour	68	17	spelt flour	96	24
cornmeal	108	27	teff flour	100	25
cornmeal, blue	100	25	triticale flour	96	24
cornstarch	116	29	wheat bran	36	9
garbanzo flour	68	17	wheat germ	40	10
gluten flour	56	14	white flour, unbleached	100	25
kamut flour	100	25	whole wheat flour	100	25
millet flour	104	26	whole wheat pastry	68	17
oat flour	60	15			

FRUIT FRESH OR COOKED (½ CUP, OR AS NOTED)

	starch calories	starch grams		starch calories	starch grams
apple (1 medium)	24	6	banana (1 medium)	24	6
applesauce	8	2	blueberries	8	2
apricots (2)	8	2	cantaloupe (¼ medium)	4	1
Asian pears (1)	16	4	carambola (1)	4	1
avocado	16	4	cherries, sweet (10)	4	1

FRUIT FRESH OR COOKED (½ CUP, OR AS NOTED) *continued*

	starch calories	starch grams		starch calories	starch grams
cranberries, raw	8	2	passion fruit (1)	8	2
grapefruit (½ medium)	8	2	peach (1 medium)	8	2
grapes, seedless	0	0	pear (1 medium)	32	8
guava (1)	24	6	persimmon, Japanese	24	6
honeydew melon (medium)	0	0	(1 large)		
			pineapple chunks	4	1
kiwifruit (2 medium)	20	5	plantain, cooked (½ cup)	80	20
kumquat (4)	0	0	plums (2 medium)	16	4
lemon (1 medium)	4	1	pomegranate (1)	24	6
lime (1 medium)	24	6	quince (1)	8	2
lychees (½ cup)	8	2	raspberries, red	4	1
mango (½ whole)	12	3	strawberries (8)	8	2
nectarine (1 medium)	12	3	tamarind (1)	4	1
orange (1 medium)	4	1	tangerine (2 medium)	16	4
papaya (½ whole)	24	6	watermelon (2 cups, diced)	4	1

GRAINS (½ CUP, COOKED)

	starch calories	starch grams		starch calories	starch grams
amaranth	88	22	oats, steel cut	70	17.5
barley, pearled	84	21	quinoa	116	29
barley, rolled flakes	52	13	rice, brown basmati	100	25
barley, whole	116	29	rice, brown long	100	25
buckwheat (kasha)	44	11	rice, white basmati	100	25
bulgur wheat	88	22	rice, white long enriched	100	25
couscous	80	20	rice, wild	72	18
granola (½ cup, dry)	104	26	rye, whole	92	23
kamut, rolled flakes	60	15	spelt, rolled flakes	104	26
kamut, whole	104	26	teff	80	20
millet	44	11	wheat, rolled flakes	64	16
oat groats	88	22	wheat, whole hard red winter	96	24
oats, rolled flakes	52	13			

NONDAIRY ALTERNATIVES—(1 CUP, OR AS NOTED)

	starch calories	starch grams		starch calories	starch grams
Almond Milk:			Rice Dream™ enriched	56	14
almond milk	0	0	Westbrae Rice Drink™	0	0
homemade	10	2.5	**Rice/Soy Milk:**		
Amasake, Grainaissance			Edenblend™	16	4
Amazake™:			**Soymilk:**		
almond	16	4	Edensoy™ Extra	20	5
almond light	4	1	Edensoy™ plain	20	6
plain	16	4	Westsoy™ plain	24	6
plain light	4	1	Westsoy™ plain light	20	5
Rice Milk:			**Soy Yogurt:**		
Eden Rice™	20	5	White Wave™ vanilla	52	13
Rice Dream™ beverage	56	14			

NUTS AND SEEDS (⅓ CUP, OR 2 TBSP. NUT BUTTER)

	starch calories	starch grams		starch calories	starch grams
almond butter	16	4	peanuts, dry roasted	32	8
almonds	28	7	pecans	16	4
Brazil nuts	20	5	pine nuts	24	6
cashew butter	28	7	pistachio nuts	28	7
cashews, roasted	48	12	pumpkin seeds, roasted	40	10
chestnuts	64	16	sesame seeds, hulled	20	5
coconut, dried	16	4	sesame seeds, whole	40	10
hazelnuts/filberts	20	5	sesame tahini	16	4
macadamia nuts	16	4	sunflower seeds	28	7
peanut butter, chunky	16	4	walnuts	20	5

PASTA (½ CUP COOKED)

	starch calories	starch grams		starch calories	starch grams
cellophane noodles	80	20	soba (40% buckwheat)	70	17.5
corn pasta	68	17	somen	92	23
egg noodles, enriched	76	19	spaghetti, spinach	68	17
fresh pasta	88	22	enriched		
sifted wheat ribbons	88	22	spaghetti, whole wheat	72	18
kamut pasta	72	18	spelt pasta	72	18
macaroni, enriched	76	19	udon noodles	66	16.5
macaroni, whole wheat	72	18	vegetable pasta, enriched	80	20
brown rice pasta	84	21			

SNACKS, MISCELLANEOUS (1 CUP, OR 18 PIECES)

	starch calories	starch grams		starch calories	starch grams
popcorn (air-popped)	24	6	tortilla chips, typical	76	19
popcorn (oil-popped)	24	6	(1 oz.)		
potato chips w/salt (17)	56	14	tortilla chips, Guiltless Gourmet™, no oil/ w/salt	88	22
potato chips, no salt (17)	56	14	tortilla chips, Guiltless Gourmet™, no oil / no salt	88	22
pretzels, typical thick Dutch	92	23			
pretzels, Newman's Own Organic™	92	23			

SPORT ENERGY BARS

	starch calories	starch grams		starch calories	starch grams
PowerBar™ apple/ cinnamon	112	28	PowerBar™ malt/nut	96	24
			Stroker™ apple oat	116	29
PowerBar™ chocolate	112	28	Stroker™ real cocoa	112	28

VEGETABLES (½ CUP RAW OR COOKED, OR AS NOTED)

	starch calories	starch grams		starch calories	starch grams
alfalfa sprouts	4	1	cucumber + peel	4	1
artichoke, steamed (1)	48	12	(⅓ medium)		
arugula, chopped	0	N/S	daikon radish, raw slices	0	0
asparagus, cooked	8	2	eggplant, cubed steamed	4	1
beets, cooked, diced	8	2	escarole, chopped	12	3
bell pepper, green	32	8	(1½ cup)		
(1 medium)			green beans, cooked	16	4
bell pepper, red	12	3	green beans, raw	12	3
(1 medium)			green onion, raw (¼ cup)	4	1
bok choy, steamed	8	2	Jerusalem artichoke, raw	44	11
broccoli (1 stalk, raw)	20	5	jicama, raw	16	4
broccoli (1 stalk,	24	6	kale, cooked	12	3
cooked)			kohlrabi, cooked	8	2
brussels sprouts,	16	4	leeks, cooked	12	3
steamed			lettuce, iceberg (1½ cups)	4	1
cabbage, cooked,	8	2	lettuce, loose, leaf	8	2
shredded			(1½ cups)		
cabbage, green, raw,	4	1	lettuce, romaine	8	2
shredded			(1½ cups)		
carrot (1 medium)	12	3	mung bean sprouts, raw	8	2
cauliflower, cooked	8	2	mung bean sprouts,	16	4
cauliflower, raw	6	1.5	stir-fried		
flowerets			mushroom, shitake,	36	9
celery (2 medium	12	3	steamed		
stalks)			mushrooms,	12	3
celery root, cooked	16	4	common		
chard, cooked	16	4	mustard greens, cooked	4	1
cilantro (¼ cup)	2	.05	okra, slices, cooked	16	4
collard greens, cooked	16	4	onion, cooked,	10	2.5
corn (1 medium ear,	84	21	chopped		
cooked)			onion, raw, chopped	8	2

VEGETABLES (½ CUP RAW OR COOKED, OR AS NOTED) *continued*

	starch calories	starch grams		starch calories	starch grams
parsley, chopped (½ cup)	4	1	red radishes (7)	4	1
pea pods (snow peas), cooked	12	3	rutabaga cube, cooked	16	4
pea pods (snow peas), raw	8	2	spaghetti squash, cooked/baked	8	2
peas, cooked from frozen	28	7	spinach, cooked	12	3
			spinach, raw (1½ cups)	12	3
peas, cooked from raw	28	7	squash, winter, baked/mashed	32	8
peas, raw	28	7	sweet potato (1 medium baked)	68	17
potato, baked (medium size)	140	35	tomato (1 medium)	0	0
potato, boiled (medium size)	104	26	tomato sauce (¼ cup)	8	2
potato, mashed w/ milk/butter	68	17	tomatoes, stewed, no salt	16	4
potato, mashed w/ milk	68	17	turnip cubes, cooked	12	3
			turnip greens, cooked	12	3
pumpkin, cooked	8	2	watercress sprigs (10)	0	0
radicchio, raw, shredded	4	1	zucchini (½ medium, raw)	8	2
			zucchini, cooked	8	2

Information extrapolated from various sources, including: United States Department of Agriculture; Wittenberg, Margaret M., *Good Food—The Comprehensive Food and Nutrition Resource*, The Crossing Press, Freedom CA, 1998; Gibney, Michael J., *Nutrition, Diet, and Health*, Cambridge University Press, Cambridge, England, 1986; Oregon Health Sciences University. See chapter notes, Appendix B.

THE GENERAL CALORIE CHART

This chart was devised especially for strategists. It's a complete calorie chart of virtually every food that is commonly eaten in America, with a very special feature: a grading system, ranking foods in relation to their value in the strategy.

The grading system assigns grades of A through F. If a food contains a high amount of starch, it gets a relatively better grade, because it's more conducive to success on the strategy. The other most important factors in determining the grade are nutrient density, amount of fiber, amount of fat, total number of calories, and presence of additives.

CALORIE CHART AND RATING SYSTEM

Food and Quantity	Starch Blocker Strategy Rating	Total Calories	Total Carbohydrate Calories	Total Protein Calories	Total Fat Calories	Fiber (g)
BEVERAGES						
Alcoholic:						
Regular Beer (12 oz)	D	146	52	4	0	1
Light Beer (12 oz)	D+	100	20	4	0	1
Gin, Rum, Vodka, Whiskey (1.5 fl oz)	D+	97	0.4	0	0	0
Coffee Liqueur (1.5 fl oz)	D	174	96	0	9	0
Red Wine (3.5 fl oz)	C	74	8	4	0	0
White Wine (3.5 fl oz)	C–	70	4	4	0	0
Nonalcoholic:						
Cola Beverage (12 oz)	F	151	156	0	0	0
Ginger Ale (12 oz)	D–	124	128	0	0	0
Orange Soda (12 oz)	F	177	184	0	0	0
Coffee (1 c)	C	2	4	4	0	1
Gatorade™ (1 c)	C+	39	44	0	0	0
Canned Grape Juice (1 c)	C	112	140	0	9	1
Kool-Aid™, w/ sugar (1 c)	C–	100	100	0	0	0
Frozen Lemonade (¾ c)	C	397	412	4	9	1
Pineapple Grapefruit (1 c)	C	117	116	4	9	0
DAIRY						
Brie (1 oz)	C	95	4	24	72	0
Cheddar, cut pieces (1 oz)	C	114	4	28	81	0
Cheddar, shredded (1 c)	C–	455	4	112	333	0

Food and Quantity	Starch Blocker Strategy Rating	Total Calories	Total Carbohydrate Calories	Total Protein Calories	Total Fat Calories	Fiber (g)
DAIRY *(continued)*						
Cottage Cheese (1 c)	C+	215	24	104	81	0
Cottage Cheese, 2% (1 c)	B	205	32	124	36	0
Cream Cheese (1 oz)	C	99	4	8	90	0
Monterey Jack (1 oz)	B	106	4	28	81	0
Mozzarella, whole milk (1 oz)	B	80	4	20	54	0
Mozzarella, skim milk (1 oz)	B	80	4	32	45	0
Parmesan, grated (1 c)	B–	455	16	168	270	0
Swiss Cheese (1 oz)	B	107	4	32	72	0
American Cheese (1 oz)	B	106	4	24	81	0
Cream, half-and-half (1 c)	C–	315	40	28	252	0
Cream, half-and-half (1 tbsp)	C–	20	4	4	18	0
Light Whipping Cream (1 c)	D	699	28	20	666	0
Light Whipping Cream (1 tbsp)	C	44	4	4	45	0
Heavy Whipping Cream (1 c)	D–	821	28	20	792	0
Heavy Whipping Cream (1 tbsp)	C–	51	4	4	54	0
Sour Cream (1 c)	C	493	40	28	432	0
Coffee Whitener:						
Frozen or Liquid (1 tbsp)	B	20	8	4	18	0
Powdered (1 tbsp)	B	11	4	4	9	0
Dessert Topping (1 tbsp)	B	11	4	4	9	0
Milk, fluid:						
Whole Milk (1 c)	C	150	44	32	72	0
2% Low-Fat Milk (1 c)	C+	121	48	32	45	0
1% Low-Fat Milk (1 c)	B	102	48	32	27	0
Skim Milk (1 c)	B	86	48	32	9	0
Buttermilk (1 c)	C+	99	48	32	18	0
Sweetened Condensed Milk (1 c)	D	982	664	96	243	0

Food and Quantity	Starch Blocker Strategy Rating	Total Calories	Total Carbohydrate Calories	Total Protein Calories	Total Fat Calories	Fiber (g)
Evaporated Skim Milk (1 c)	C+	200	116	76	9	0
Goat Milk (1 c)	B	168	44	36	90	0
Kefir (1 c)	B+	122	36	36	45	0
Eggnog (1 c)	B–	342	136	40	171	0
Instant Breakfast:						
Envelope, dry powder only (1)	B	130	92	28	0	0
Prepared w/ whole milk (1 c)	B–	280	136	60	72	0
Milk Shakes:						
Chocolate (1¼ c)	D	360	232	40	99	1
Vanilla (1¼ c)	D	314	204	40	72	1
Ice Cream, Vanilla (11% fat):						
Hardened (1 c)	D	269	128	20	126	0
Soft Serve (1 c)	D	377	152	28	198	0
Pudding:						
Canned Pudding:						
Chocolate (1)	D	205	120	12	99	1
Vanilla (1)	D	220	132	8	90	0
Prepared with whole milk:						
Chocolate, instant (1 c)	D	310	216	32	72	1
Vanilla, instant (1 c)	D	150	108	16	36	0
Soy Milk (1 c)	C	79	16	28	45	0
Yogurt, low fat:						
Fruit added (1 c)	C+	231	172	40	18	1
Plain (1 c)	C+	144	64	48	27	0
Eggs:						
Whole, without shell (1)	B	75	4	24	45	0
Egg White (1)	B+	17	4	16	0	0
Scrambled w/milk and margarine (1)	B	100	4	28	63	0
FATS AND OILS						
Butter:						
Stick (½ c)	D	813	4	4	828	0
1 Tablespoon	C+	100	4	4	108	0
Vegetable Shortening (1 tbsp)	B	15	0	0	117	0

Food and Quantity	Starch Blocker Strategy Rating	Total Calories	Total Carbohydrate Calories	Total Protein Calories	Total Fat Calories	Fiber (g)
FATS AND OILS *(continued)*						
Margarine:						
Imitation, 40% fat (1 tbsp)	F	50	0.4	0.4	54	0
Regular, 80% fat (1 tbsp)	F	100	4	4	99	0
Spread, 60% fat (1 tbsp)	F	75	0	0.4	81	0
Oils:						
Canola (1 tbsp)	C	125	0	0	126	0
Corn (1 tbsp)	C	125	0	0	126	0
Olive (1 tbsp)	B+	125	0	0	126	0
Peanut (1 tbsp)	C	125	0	0	126	0
Soybean (1 tbsp)	B	125	0	0	126	0
Sunflower (1 tbsp)	C	125	0	0	126	0
Salad Dressings:						
Blue Cheese (1 tbsp)	C	75	4	4	72	1
French (1 tbsp)	C	85	4	0.4	81	1
Italian (1 tbsp)	C+	80	4	4	81	1
Thousand Island (1 tbsp)	C	60	8	4	54	1
Mayonnaise:						
Regular (1 tbsp)	C–	100	4	4	99	0
Imitation (1 tbsp)	D	35	8	0	27	0
Tartar Sauce (1 tbsp)	C	74	4	4	72	1
FRUITS						
Apples:						
2¾" diameter (1)	A	80	84	4	9	3
3¼" diameter (1)	A	125	128	4	9	5
Applesauce, unsweetened (1 c)	B+	106	112	4	9	4
Applesauce, sweetened (1 c)	B	195	204	4	9	4
Apricots, raw (3)	A	51	48	4	9	2
Avocados (1)	B–	340	108	20	243	29
Bananas (1)	B	105	108	4	9	2
Blackberries (1 c)	A	74	72	4	9	10
Blueberries, fresh (1 c)	A	82	84	4	9	4
Cherries, canned (1 c)	B–	90	88	8	9	3
Cranberry Sauce (1 c)	B–	149	432	4	9	6

Food and Quantity	Starch Blocker Strategy Rating	Total Calories	Total Carbohydrate Calories	Total Protein Calories	Total Fat Calories	Fiber (g)
Grapefruit (.5)	A	37	36	4	9	2
Grapes, raw, seedless (10)	A	35	36	4	9	1
Kiwifruit (1)	A	46	44	4	9	3
Lemons (1)	A	17	20	4	9	1
Mangoes (1)	A	135	140	4	9	7
Cantaloupe (.5)	A	94	88	8	9	3
Honeydew (1 slice)	A	45	48	4	9	1
Nectarines (1)	A	67	64	4	9	3
Oranges (1)	A	60	60	4	9	3
Peaches, peeled (1)	A–	37	40	4	9	2
Pears, cored:						
Bartlett (1)	A	98	100	4	9	5
Bosc (1)	A	85	84	4	9	4
D'Anjou (1)	A	120	120	4	9	6
Pineapple (1 c)	A	76	76	4	9	2
Plantain, w/out peel (1 c)	A	181	188	8	9	7
Plums (1)	A	36	36	4	9	1
Prunes, dried, pitted (10)	A	201	212	8	9	8
Raisins, seedless (1 c)	A	435	460	20	9	9
Raisin package (.5 oz)	A	41	44	4	0.9	1
Raspberries, fresh (1 c)	A	60	56	4	9	8
Rhubarb, cooked w/ sugar (1 c)	B	279	300	4	9	5
Strawberries, fresh (1 c)	A	45	44	4	9	4
Strawberries, frozen, sweetened (10 oz)	B–	273	296	8	9	6
Tangerines, no peel (1)	A	37	36	4	9	2
Watermelon (1 piece)	A	152	140	12	18	2
BAKED GOODS						
Bagels, plain (1)	D	180	140	28	9	1
Biscuits:						
From home recipe (1)	D	100	52	8	45	1
From mix (1)	D–	94	56	8	27	1
Breads:						
Cracked wheat (1 slice)	B	65	52	8	9	1
French/Vienna (1 slice)	C	100	72	12	9	1
Italian, enriched (1 slice)	C	83	68	12	9	1
Mixed grain (1 slice)	C+	65	48	8	9	2

Food and Quantity	Starch Blocker Strategy Rating	Total Calories	Total Carbohydrate Calories	Total Protein Calories	Total Fat Calories	Fiber (g)
BAKED GOODS *(continued)*						
Breads:						
Oatmeal (1 slice)	C+	65	48	8	9	1
Pita pocket bread (1 slice)	B	165	132	24	9	1
Pumpernickel (1 slice)	B	80	60	12	9	2
Raisin (1 slice)	C	68	52	8	9	1
Rye (1 slice)	C+	65	48	8	9	2
Wheat (1 slice)	C	65	48	8	9	1
White, enriched (1 slice)	C–	65	48	8	9	1
Whole wheat (1 slice)	C	70	52	12	9	2
Cakes, prepared from mixes:						
Angel food (1 piece)	D	125	116	12	9	1
Boston cream pie (1 piece)	F	260	176	12	72	1
Coffee cake (1 piece)	D	230	152	20	63	2
Gingerbread (1 piece)	C–	174	128	8	36	2
Yellow w/ frosting (1 piece)	D–	235	160	12	72	1
Fruitcake (1 piece)	D	165	100	8	63	2
Cheese puffs/Cheetos™ (1 oz)	D	158	56	8	90	1
Cookies, made w/ enriched flour:						
Brownies w/ nuts (1)	D	95	44	4	54	1
Chocolate chip cookies (4)	D	185	104	8	99	1
Fig bars (4)	D	210	164	8	36	3
Oatmeal raisin cookies (4)	C–	245	144	12	90	1
Peanut butter cookies (4)	D	245	100	8	126	1
Sugar cookies (4)	D	235	124	8	108	1
Vanilla wafers (10)	D	185	116	8	63	1
Corn chips (1 oz)	D	155	64	8	81	1
Crackers:						
Cheese crackers (10)	C–	50	20	4	27	1
Crackers w/ peanut butter (4)	C–	150	76	16	72	1
Graham crackers (2)	C	60	44	4	9	1

Food and Quantity	Starch Blocker Strategy Rating	Total Calories	Total Carbohydrate Calories	Total Protein Calories	Total Fat Calories	Fiber (g)
Melba toast™, plain (1 piece)	C+	20	16	4	9	1
Saltine™ crackers (4)	C+	50	36	4	9	1
Wheat crackers, thin (4)	C+	35	20	4	9	1
Croissants (1)	C–	235	108	20	108	1
Apple crisp (1)	C	146	100	4	45	1
Cherry cobbler (1 piece)	C–	199	136	8	54	1
Doughnuts:						
Cake type, plain (1)	D	210	100	8	108	1
Yeast-leavened glaze (1)	D	235	104	16	117	1
English muffins (1)	C	140	104	20	9	2
Muffins: 2¼" by 1½":						
Blueberry (1)	C	135	80	12	45	2
Bran, wheat (1)	C+	125	76	12	54	3
Cornmeal (1)	C–	145	84	12	45	2
Pancakes, 4"diam:						
Buckwheat, from mix (1)	C	55	24	8	18	1
Plain, from home recipe (1)	C	60	36	8	18	1
Piecrust, w /vegetable shortening (1)	C–	900	316	44	540	4
Pies, 9" diameter:						
Apple pie (1 piece)	C+	405	240	16	162	3
Banana cream (1 piece)	D	319	188	24	117	2
Blueberry pie (1 piece)	C+	380	220	16	153	4
Cherry pie (1 piece)	C+	410	244	16	162	2
Chocolate cream (1 piece)	D	311	168	28	117	1
Peach pie (1 piece)	C+	405	244	16	153	3
Pumpkin pie (1 piece)	C	367	204	36	144	5
Pretzels, w/ enriched flour:						
Thin sticks (10)	B	10	8	4	9	1
Dutch twist (1)	B–	65	52	8	9	1
Thin twist (10)	B–	240	192	24	18	2

Food and Quantity	Starch Blocker Strategy Rating	Total Calories	Total Carbohydrate Calories	Total Protein Calories	Total Fat Calories	Fiber (g)
BAKED GOODS *(continued)*						
Rolls and buns, enriched:						
Hot dog buns (1)	C–	115	80	12	18	1
Hamburger buns (1)	C–	129	92	16	18	1
Submarine/Hoagie rolls (1)	C–	400	288	44	72	2
Tortilla chips:						
Plain (1 oz)	C	139	68	8	72	1
Nacho flavor (1 oz)	C	139	72	8	63	1
Taco flavor (1 oz)	C	140	72	12	63	1
Tortillas:						
Corn, enriched, 6" (1)	C+	65	52	8	9	2
Flour, 8" (1)	C	105	76	12	27	1
Flour, 10.5" (1)	C	168	124	16	36	2
Taco shells (1)		59	36	4	18	1
Waffles, 7"diameter:						
From home recipe (1)	C+	245	104	28	117	1
From mix, egg, milk (1)	C	205	108	28	72	1
GRAIN PRODUCTS						
Barley, pearled:						
Dry, uncooked (1 c)	B	700	632	64	18	31
Cooked (1 c)	B+	193	176	16	9	4
Cereals, hot, cooked:						
Grits, regular & quick (1 c)	B+	146	124	16	9	5
Grits, instant, from packet (1 c)	B	80	72	8	9	3
Cream of Wheat, instant (1 c)	B	140	116	16	9	3
Cream of Wheat, packet (1 c)	B	100	84	12	9	2
Oatmeal, regular, instant (1 c)	B	145	100	24	18	4
Oatmeal, plain, from packet (.75 c)	B	104	72	16	18	3
Oatmeal, flavored, from packet (.75 c)	B	160	124	20	18	3

Food and Quantity	Starch Blocker Strategy Rating	Total Calories	Total Carbohydrate Calories	Total Protein Calories	Total Fat Calories	Fiber (g)
Breakfast cereals:						
All-Bran™ (⅓ c)	A	70	88	16	9	9
Apple Jacks™ (1 c)	B	110	104	8	9	1
Bran Chex™ (1 c)	B–	156	156	20	9	9
Cap'n Crunch™ (1 c)	C	156	120	8	27	1
Cheerios™ (1 c)	B	89	64	12	9	2
Corn Chex™ (1 c)	B	111	100	8	9	1
Corn Flakes™ (1.25 c)	B	110	96	8	9	1
Cracklin' Oat Bran™ (1 c)	C	229	164	24	81	9
Froot Loops™ (1 c)	C–	111	100	8	9	1
Frosted Mini-Wheats™ (4)	C–	111	104	12	9	2
Fruit & Fiber™, w/ apples (1 c)	B	180	176	24	18	8
Fruity Pebbles™ (⅞ c)	C	113	96	4	18	1
Grape-Nuts™ (1 c)	B+	420	368	48	9	10
Life™ cereal (1 c)	B	162	128	32	9	1
Raisin Bran™, Kellogg's (1 c)	B	158	148	20	9	6
Rice Krispies™ (1 c)	B	112	100	8	9	1
Shredded Wheat™ (¾ c)	B+	115	100	12	9	4
Wheaties™ (1 c)	B	101	92	12	9	3
Cornmeal:						
Whole-ground, dry (1 c)	B+	442	376	40	36	13
Degermed, enriched, dry (1 c)	B	505	428	48	18	10
Macaroni, enriched (1 c)	B–	197	160	28	9	2
Noodles:						
Egg noodles, cooked (1 c)	B	213	160	32	18	4
Chow mein, dry (1 c)	B	237	104	16	126	2
Spinach noodles, dry (3.5 oz)	B+	372	300	52	18	7
Popcorn:						
Air popped, plain (1 c)	B	30	24	4	9	1
Veg. oil, salted (1 c)	B–	55	24	4	27	1
Sugar-syrup coated (1 c)	C	135	120	8	9	1

Food and Quantity	Starch Blocker Strategy Rating	Total Calories	Total Carbohydrate Calories	Total Protein Calories	Total Fat Calories	Fiber (g)
GRAIN PRODUCTS *(continued)*						
Rice:						
Brown rice, cooked (1 c)	A	217	180	20	18	3
White, enriched, all types:	B					
Regular/long grain, dry (1 c)	B	675	592	52	9	2
Regular/long grain, cooked (1 c)	B	264	228	24	9	1
Instant, no salt (1 c)	B	162	140	12	9	1
Wild rice, cooked (1 c)	B	166	140	16	9	3
Rye flour, medium (1 c)	B	361	316	40	18	15
Spaghetti, cooked:						
Enriched, w/out salt (1 c)	B	197	160	28	9	2
Whole wheat, cooked (1 c)	B+	174	148	28	9	5
Wheat germ:						
Raw (1 c)	A	360	208	92	90	12
Toasted (1 c)	A	432	224	132	108	16
Whole-grain wheat (⅓ c)	A	28	28	4	9	1
All-purpose white flour (1 c)	C	455	380	52	9	3
Cake/pastry flour (1 c)	C	348	300	32	9	3
Self-rising, enriched (1 c)	C	442	372	48	9	3
Whole wheat (1 c)	B	407	348	64	18	15
MEATS: FISH & SHELLFISH						
Bass, baked or broiled (3.5 oz)	A	125	0	96	36	0
Clams:						
Raw meat only (3 oz)	A	63	8	44	9	1
Canned, drained (3 oz)	A	126	16	88	18	0
Steamed, meat only (20)	A	133	20	92	18	1

Food and Quantity	Starch Blocker Strategy Rating	Total Calories	Total Carbohydrate Calories	Total Protein Calories	Total Fat Calories	Fiber (g)
Dungeness crab, cooked (¾ c)	A	85	4	72	18	0
Crab, imitation (3 oz)	A	87	36	40	9	0
Herring, pickled (3oz)	A	223	32	48	135	0
Lobster, cooked (1 c)	A	142	8	120	9	0
Oysters:						
Raw, Eastern (1 c)	A	170	40	72	54	0
Raw, Pacific (1 c)	A	200	48	92	54	0
Eastern, breaded, fried (6)	C	173	40	32	99	1
Pacific, simmered (3.5 oz)	A	135	28	76	18	0
Pollack, baked or broiled (3.5 oz)	A	96	0	80	9	0
Salmon:						
Canned pink, solids & liquid (3 oz)	A	118	0	68	45	0
Broiled or baked (3 oz)	A	183	0	92	81	0
Smoked (3 oz)	A	99	0	64	36	0
Scallops, breaded (6)	B	200	36	68	90	1
Shrimp:						
Cooked, boiled, 18 large (3.5 oz)	A	99	0	84	9	0
Canned, drained (⅔ c)	A	102	4	80	18	0
Fried, 4 large = 30g (12)	C	218	40	76	99	1
Snapper, baked or broiled (3.5 oz)	A	128	0	104	18	0
Trout (3 oz)	A	129	4	88	36	0
Tuna:						
Canned, oil pack (3 oz)	C	163	0	100	63	0
Canned, water pack (3 oz)	A	111	0	100	9	0
Raw (3.5 oz)	A	144	0	92	45	0

MEATS: BEEF, LAMP, PORK, & OTHERS

Beef, cooked:
Braised, simmered, pot roasted, choice chuck blade:

Food and Quantity	Starch Blocker Strategy Rating	Total Calories	Total Carbohydrate Calories	Total Protein Calories	Total Fat Calories	Fiber (g)
Lean and fat (3 oz)	C–	309	0	88	216	0
Lean only (3 oz)	B	224	0	104	108	0

Food and Quantity	Starch Blocker Strategy Rating	Total Calories	Total Carbohydrate Calories	Total Protein Calories	Total Fat Calories	Fiber (g)
MEATS: BEEF, LAMP, PORK, & OTHERS *(continued)*						
Ground beef, 3 × ⅝":						
Extra lean, 16% fat						
(3 oz)	B+	225	0	96	117	0
Lean, 21% fat (3 oz)	B	238	0	96	135	0
Roast, oven cooked, no liquid added:						
Lean and fat (3 oz)	C	348	0	76	270	0
Lean only (3 oz)	B	248	0	92	153	0
Steak, broiled, relatively lean:						
Lean and fat (3 oz)	C	229	0	96	126	0
Lean only (3 oz)	B	172	0	104	63	0
Lamb, domestic, cooked:						
Chop, loin, broiled,						
w/ fat (2.3 oz)	C	201	0	64	135	0
Chop, loin, broiled,						
lean (1.6 oz)	B	100	0	56	45	0
Leg, roasted, w/ fat						
(3 oz)	C	219	0	88	126	0
Leg, roasted, lean (3 oz)	B	162	0	96	63	0
Rib, roasted, w/ fat (3 oz)	C	305	0	72	225	0
Rib, roasted, lean (3 oz)	B	163	0	88	72	0
Pork, cured, cooked:						
Bacon, medium						
slices (3)	D	109	4	24	81	0
Breakfast strips,						
cooked (3)	D	156	4	40	117	0
Ham, roasted, w/						
fat (3 oz)	D	207	0	72	126	0
Ham, roasted lean						
only (3 oz)	B	133	0	84	45	0
Chops, loin, 3 per lb w/ bone:						
Braised, w/ fat (1)	C–	261	0	76	180	0
Braised, lean only (1)	B	150	0	72	72	0
Broiled, w/ fat (3.1 oz)	C	275	0	96	171	0
Broiled, lean only						
(2.5 oz)	B	166	0	92	72	0
Spareribs, cooked w/						
bone (6.25 oz)	C	703	0	204	486	0
Venison, roasted						
(3.5 oz)	B	158	0	120	27	0

Food and Quantity	Starch Blocker Strategy Rating	Total Calories	Total Carbohydrate Calories	Total Protein Calories	Total Fat Calories	Fiber (g)
MEATS: POULTRY						
Chicken, fried, batter dipped:						
Breast, 5.6 oz w/ bones (1)	C	364	52	140	171	1
Drumstick, 2.6 oz w/ bones (1)	C	193	24	64	99	1
Thigh (1)	C	238	32	76	126	1
Wing (1)	C	159	20	40	99	1
Chicken, roasted:						
Dark meat (1 c)	B+	286	0	152	126	0
Light meat (1 c)	B+	242	0	172	54	0
Breast, w/out skin (.5)	A	142	0	108	27	0
Drumstick (1)	B+	76	0	52	90	0
Thigh (1)	B+	153	0	64	90	0
Turkey, roasted, meat only:						
Dark meat (3 oz)	A	159	0	96	54	0
Light meat (3 oz)	A	133	0	100	27	0
Ground turkey, cooked (3.5 oz)	A	229	0	96	126	0
Breast, barbecued (1 oz)	A	40	0	24	9	0
MEATS: SAUSAGES AND LUNCHMEATS						
Beef bologna (1)	F	75	4	12	63	0
Pork bologna (1)	F	57	4	16	45	0
Brown-and-serve sausage (1)	F	50	4	8	45	0
Frankfurters:						
Beef, large link (1)	D	184	4	24	153	0
Beef and pork, large (1)	F	183	4	24	153	0
Ham lunchmeat, regular (2)	F	103	8	40	54	0
Kielbasa sausage (1)	D	81	4	12	63	0
Pepperoni sausage, slices (4)	D	149	12	28	108	1
Salami:						
Pork and beef (2 pieces)	D	143	4	32	99	0
Turkey (2 pieces)	C	111	4	36	72	0

Food and Quantity	Starch Blocker Strategy Rating	Total Calories	Total Carbohydrate Calories	Total Protein Calories	Total Fat Calories	Fiber (g)
MEATS: SAUSAGES AND LUNCHMEATS *(continued)*						
Salami:						
Dry, beef and pork (2 pieces)	D	85	4	20	63	0
Summer sausage (1 piece)	D	80	4	16	63	0
MIXED DISHES AND FAST FOODS						
Beef stew w/ vegetables (1 c)	B	194	72	56	72	1
Chicken and noodles (1 c)	B	365	104	88	162	1
Chicken salad w/ celery (½ c)	B	266	4	44	225	1
Chili w/ beans, canned (1 c)	C+	286	120	60	126	8
Coleslaw (1 c)	B	84	60	8	27	2
Egg salad (1 c)	B	438	12	76	351	1
Lasagna, w/ meat (1 piece)	B–	398	120	104	180	2
Lasagna, w/out meat (1 piece)	B–	316	120	80	126	2
Macaroni and cheese (1 c)	C	430	160	68	198	1
Meat loaf, beef (1 piece)	B	193	16	64	108	1
Spaghetti:						
with cheese, homemade	B–	260	148	36	81	3
with cheese, canned	C	190	156	24	18	3
Tuna salad	B+	383	76	132	171	2
Fast foods:						
Burrito, beef and bean (1)	C–	390	160	84	162	5
Burrito, bean (1)	C	322	188	52	90	8
Cheeseburger, regular (1)	C–	300	112	60	135	1
Corn dog (1)	C–	330	108	40	180	1
Fish sandwich, w/ cheese (1)	C	420	156	64	207	1

Food and Quantity	Starch Blocker Strategy Rating	Total Calories	Total Carbohydrate Calories	Total Protein Calories	Total Fat Calories	Fiber (g)
Hamburger w/ bun (1)	C	245	112	48	99	1
Cheese pizza (1 piece)	C	290	156	60	81	2
Sandwiches, on white bread:						
Bacon, lettuce, and tomato (1)	D	333	120	44	171	2
Cheese sandwich, grilled (1)	D+	399	112	68	216	1
Egg salad sandwich (1)	C–	325	112	36	171	1
Ham sandwich (1)	D	262	112	64	81	1
Ham and cheese sandwich (1)	D	369	116	88	162	1
Peanut butter and jam (1)	C–	347	180	48	135	3
Roast beef sandwich (1)	C	286	112	68	99	1
Tuna salad sandwich (1)	C+	309	84	52	126	2
Turkey sandwich (1)	C+	259	116	64	81	1
Taco, corn tortilla, beef (1)	C+	207	40	56	117	1
Tostada:						
w/ refried beans (1)	C	212	104	40	81	7
w/ beans and beef (1)	C+	332	80	72	189	4
w/ beans and chicken (1)	C+	249	76	76	99	4
Vegetarian foods:						
Proteena (1 piece)	B	160	20	32	108	1
Vege-burger (1 piece)	B	130	20	56	54	1
Breakfast links (½ c)	B	110	16	88	9	1
NUTS, SEEDS, AND PRODUCTS						
Almonds:						
Dry roasted, salted (1 c)	B–	810	132	92	639	18
Whole, dried unsalted (1 c)	B	837	116	112	666	17
Cashew, roasted, w/ salt (1 c)	B–	787	180	84	567	8
Coconut:						
Raw piece (1 piece)	B	159	28	8	135	5
Shredded (1 c)	B	283	48	12	243	9

Food and Quantity	Starch Blocker Strategy Rating	Total Calories	Total Carbohydrate Calories	Total Protein Calories	Total Fat Calories	Fiber (g)
NUTS, SEEDS, AND PRODUCTS *(continued)*						
Mixed nuts:						
Dry roasted, salted (1 c)	C+	814	140	96	630	12
Oil roasted, salted (1 c)	C	876	120	96	720	13
Peanuts:						
Oil roasted, salted (1 c)	C	837	108	152	639	13
Dried, unsalted (1 c)	C+	827	96	152	648	13
Peanut butter (1 tbsp)	B–	94	12	16	72	1
Pistachios, dried, shelled (1 oz)	B	164	28	24	126	1
Sesame seeds, dried (¼ c)	B	221	16	40	189	6
Sunflower seeds, dry (¼ c)	B	205	28	32	162	2
Sunflower seeds, oil (¼ c)	B–	208	20	28	171	2
English walnuts (1 c)	B	770	88	68	666	7
SWEETENERS AND SWEETS						
Cake frosting:						
Canned, average all types (2.5 tbsp)	D	160	96	0	63	0
Prepared from mix (2.5 tbsp)	D	167	112	0	54	0
Milk chocolate, plain (1 oz)	D	145	64	8	81	1
Semisweet chocolate chips (1 c)	D	860	388	28	549	5
Fudge, chocolate (1 oz)	D	115	84	4	27	2
Hard candy, all flavors (1 oz)	D	109	112	0	0	0
M&M's™, plain (48 g)	D	237	132	12	90	1
Mars™ bar (1)	D	240	120	16	99	1
Milky Way™ (1)	D	260	172	12	81	1
Reese's™ peanut butter cup (2)	D	240	88	24	126	2
Snickers™ (1)	D	290	148	28	126	2
Honey (1 tbsp)	C	65	68	0.4	0	0
Marshmallows (4)	D	90	92	0	0	0
Popsicles (1)	D	70	72	0	0	0

Food and Quantity	Starch Blocker Strategy Rating	Total Calories	Total Carbohydrate Calories	Total Protein Calories	Total Fat Calories	Fiber (g)
Sugars:						
Brown sugar (1 c)	D	820	848	0	0	0
White sugar, granulated (1 c)	D	770	796	0	0	0
White sugar, powdered, sifted (1 c)	D+	385	396	0	0	0
Syrups:						
Chocolate fudge (2 tbsp)	D	125	84	8	45	1
Molasses, blackstrap (2 tbsp)	C	85	88	0	0	0
Pancake table syrup (2 tbsp)	D	244	256	0	0	0
VEGETABLES AND LEGUMES						
Alfalfa seeds, sprouted (1 c)	A	10	4	4	9	1
Artichokes (1)	A	60	52	16	9	10
Asparagus, green, cooked (4)	A	15	12	8	9	1
Beans:						
Garbanzo beans (1 c)	B	269	180	60	36	11
Great northern beans, cooked (1 c)	B	210	148	60	9	11
Kidney beans, canned (1 c)	B	216	156	52	9	19
Navy beans, cooked (1 c)	B	259	192	64	9	16
Pinto beans, cooked (1 c)	B	235	176	56	9	20
Refried beans, canned (1 c)	C	270	188	64	27	22
Soybeans, cooked (1 c)	B+	398	68	116	135	5
Snap/green beans, raw (1 c)	A	44	40	8	9	3
Bean sprouts, stir-fried (1 c)	A	62	52	20	9	3
Beets (2)	A	31	28	4	0.9	2
Beets, canned (½ c)	B+	74	76	4	9	2
Broccoli, raw, chopped (1 c)	A	24	20	12	9	3

Food and Quantity	Starch Blocker Strategy Rating	Total Calories	Total Carbohydrate Calories	Total Protein Calories	Total Fat Calories	Fiber (g)
VEGETABLES AND LEGUMES *(continued)*						
Brussels sprouts, raw (1 c)	A	60	56	24	9	6
Cabbage, common (1 c)	A	16	16	4	9	2
Carrots:						
Raw (1)	A	31	28	4	9	2
Cooked from raw (½ c)	A	35	32	4	9	3
Carrot juice (½ c)	A	49	44	4	9	2
Cauliflower, from frozen (½ c)	A–	34	28	12	9	3
Celery, raw (1)	A	6	4	4	0.9	1
Collards, from frozen (1 c)	A	63	56	12	9	6
Corn:						
From raw, on cob (1)	A	83	76	12	9	3
Kernels, from frozen (½ c)	A–	67	68	8	0.9	3
Canned, cream style (½ c)	B	93	92	8	9	2
Whole kernel, vacuum pack (1 c)	A	166	164	20	9	3
Cucumbers, w/ peel (6 pieces)	A	4	4	4	0.9	1
Eggplant, cooked (1 c)	A	45	44	4	9	6
Jerusalem artichokes, raw (1 c)	A	114	104	12	0.9	2
Leeks, raw, chopped (1 c)	A	63	60	8	9	2
Lentils, from dry (1 c)	A	230	160	72	9	10
Lettuce:						
Iceberg/crisp, head (1)	A	70	44	20	9	9
Wedge (¼ of head)	A	18	12	4	9	2
Loose leaf, chopped (1 c)	A	10	8	4	9	1
Romaine, chopped (1 c)	A	9	4	4	9	1
Mushrooms, raw (½ c)	A	9	8	4	9	1

Food and Quantity	Starch Blocker Strategy Rating	Total Calories	Total Carbohydrate Calories	Total Protein Calories	Total Fat Calories	Fiber (g)
Onions:						
Raw, chopped (1 c)	A	61	56	8	9	3
Raw, sliced (1 c)	A	44	40	4	9	2
Spring onions, white only (1 c)	A	50	40	4	9	3
Onion rings (2)	B	81	32	4	45	1
Parsnips, sliced, cooked (1 c)	A	125	120	8	9	5
Peas, cooked:	A					
Black-eyed Peas:	A					
From dry, drained (1 c)	A	198	144	52	9	21
From fresh, drained (1 c)	A	160	132	20	9	12
From frozen, drained (1 c)	A–	224	160	56	9	14
Green Peas, canned (1 c)	A–	118	88	32	9	8
Split, green, from dry (1 c)	A	231	164	64	9	10
Hot green chili, canned (½ c)	A–	17	16	4	0.9	1
Jalapeños, canned (½ c)	A–	17	12	4	9	2
Peppers, sweet, green (1)	A	20	20	4	9	1
Peppers, sweet, red (½ c)	A	19	20	4	9	1
Potatoes:						
Baked (1)	B	220	204	20	9	5
Boiled (1)	B+	119	108	12	9	2
French fries 2–3 1/2" long, frozen:						
Oven heated (10)	B	111	68	8	36	1
Fried in vegetable oil (10)	C	158	80	8	72	1
Hashed brown, frozen (1 c)	C	340	176	20	162	3
Mashed Potatoes (1 c):						
Home recipe w/ milk and margarine	C–	222	140	16	171	3

Food and Quantity	Starch Blocker Strategy Rating	Total Calories	Total Carbohydrate Calories	Total Protein Calories	Total Fat Calories	Fiber (g)
VEGETABLES AND LEGUMES *(continued)*						
Mashed Potatoes (1 c):						
Flakes: water, milk, margarine	D	239	112	16	117	2
Potato products, prepared:						
Au gratin, dry mix (1 c)	C	228	128	24	90	4
Scalloped, dry mix (1 c)	C	228	124	20	99	3
Potato chips (14 chips = 1 oz)	C	148	60	8	90	1
Pumpkin, canned (1 c)	B	83	80	12	9	5
Red radishes (10)	A	7	8	4	9	1
Soybean products:						
Miso (½ c)	A	283	156	64	72	7
Tofu (½ c)	A	94	8	40	54	2
Spinach, raw, chopped (1 c)	A	12	8	8	9	2
Squash, summer varieties (1 c)	A	36	32	8	9	3
Squash, winter varieties (1 c)	A	96	84	8	18	7
Zucchini (1 c)	A	29	28	4	0.9	4
Acorn squash, baked (1 c)	A	137	144	12	9	7
Spaghetti squash, baked (1 c)	A	45	40	4	9	4
Succotash, from frozen (1 c)	A	158	136	28	18	9
Sweet potatoes (1)	B	160	148	8	9	5
Tomatoes:						
Raw, whole (1)	A	26	24	4	9	2
Cooked from raw (1 c)	A	65	56	12	9	4
Tomato juice, canned (1 c)	B	42	40	8	9	2
Tomato paste (1 c)	B	220	196	40	18	11
Tomato puree (1 c)	B	102	100	16	9	6
Tomato sauce 1 c)	B	74	72	12	9	4
Watercress, fresh, chopped (½ c)	A	2	4	4	9	1

Food and Quantity	Starch Blocker Strategy Rating	Total Calories	Total Carbohydrate Calories	Total Protein Calories	Total Fat Calories	Fiber (g)
Miscellaneous						
Baking powder (1 tbsp)	C	5	4	0	0	0
Baking soda (1 tbsp)	C	0	0	0	0	0
Carob flour (1 c)	C	185	368	20	9	34
Catsup (1 c)	C	255	268	16	9	4
Chocolate, baking, unsweetened (1 oz)	C	145	28	16	135	4
Cornstarch (1 tbsp)	C	20	20	0.4	0.9	0.1
Cinnamon (1 tsp)	C	6	8	4	0.9	1
Hummus (1 c)	A	420	200	132	189	4
Olives, green (10)	A	45	4	4	54	1
Pickles:						
Dill, medium (1)	C	12	12	4	9	1
Sweet, medium (1)	C	41	44	4	0.9	1
Salsa, from recipe (¾ c)	B	79	36	8	45	3
Salt (1 tsp)	D	0	0	0	0	0
SOUPS, SAUCES, AND GRAVIES						
Soups:						
Canned condensed:						
Cream of celery (1 c)	C–	180	72	12	99	1
Cream of chicken (1 c)	C–	233	76	28	135	1
Cream of mushroom (1 c)	C–	257	76	16	171	1
Onion (1 c)	B	114	64	32	27	1
Prepared with whole milk:						
Clam chowder, New England (1 c)	C	163	68	36	63	1
Tomato (1 c)	C	160	88	24	54	1
Prepared with water:						
Bean with bacon (1 c)	C+	173	92	32	54	3
Chicken noodle (1 c)	B	75	36	16	18	1
Chili beef soup (1 c)	B	169	88	28	63	1
Split pea w/ ham (1 c)	B–	189	112	40	36	1
Sauces:						
Dry mix, w/ milk:						
Cheese sauce (1 c)	C–	305	92	64	153	1
Hollandaise (1 c)	C–	240	56	20	117	0

Food and Quantity	Starch Blocker Strategy Rating	Total Calories	Total Carbohydrate Calories	Total Protein Calories	Total Fat Calories	Fiber (g)
SOUPS, SAUCES, AND GRAVIES *(continued)*						
Sauces:						
Ready to serve:						
Barbecue sauce (1 tbsp)	B	10	8	4	9	1
Soy sauce (1 tbsp)	B	9	8	4	0	0
Spaghetti sauce, canned:						
Plain (1)	B–	272	160	20	108	3
With meat (¾ c)	B–	220	108	32	90	1
With mushrooms (¾ c)	B–	162	36	8	45	2
Teriyaki sauce (1 tbsp)	B	15	12	4	9	0
Gravies:						
Canned:						
Beef (1 c)	C	123	44	36	45	1
Chicken (1 c)	C+	189	52	20	126	1
Mushrooms (1 c)	C+	120	52	12	54	1
From dry mix:						
Brown (1 c)	C	75	52	8	18	1
Chicken (1 c)	C	85	56	12	18	1
POPULAR FAST-FOOD RESTAURANTS						
Arby's™:						
Bac'n' Cheddar, deluxe (1)	D	532	140	116	297	1
Roast beef sandwiches:						
Regular (1)	D	353	128	88	135	1
Junior (1)	D	218	84	52	639	1
Arby's™:						
Roast beef sandwiches:						
Super (1)	D	529	184	132	261	1
Deluxe (1)	D	486	172	104	207	1
Beef 'n' Cheddar (1)	D–	451	168	100	180	1
Chicken sandwiches:						
Chicken breast sandwich (1)	B	489	192	92	234	1
Chicken club sandwich (1)	B–	513	160	128	261	1
Baked Potatoes:						
Plain (1)	B	240	200	24	18	6

Food and Quantity	Starch Blocker Strategy Rating	Total Calories	Total Carbohydrate Calories	Total Protein Calories	Total Fat Calories	Fiber (g)
Sour cream and butter (1)	C–	463	212	32	225	6
Broccoli and cheese (1)	C	417	340	44	162	6
Taco (1)	C	619	292	92	243	6
Burger King™:						
Croissant sandwiches:						
egg, bacon, and cheese (1)	D	335	80	60	216	1
egg, ham, and cheese (1)	D	335	80	72	180	1
Whopper sandwiches:						
Whopper (1)	D	640	168	108	369	1
Double beef (1)	D	850	208	184	468	1
Whopper, Junior (1)	D	370	124	60	153	1
Hamburger (1)	D	275	116	60	108	1
Cheeseburger (1)	D	317	120	68	135	1
Chicken Sandwich (1)	C–	688	224	104	360	1
Chicken tenders (1)	C	204	40	80	90	0
Whaler fish sandwich (1)	C–	488	180	76	243	1
French fries, regular (1 srv)	C	227	96	12	117	1
Onion rings, regular (1 srv)	C	274	68	16	144	1
Apple pie (1)	C–	305	176	12	108	1
Cherry pie (1)	C–	357	220	16	117	1
Pecan pie (1)	C–	459	260	20	180	1
Dairy Queen™:						
Ice cream cone, regular (1)	C	240	152	24	63	0
Ice cream cone, dipped, regular (1)	C–	340	168	24	144	1
Sundae, regular (1)	D	310	224	20	72	1
Banana split (1)	D	540	412	36	99	1
Peanut buster parfait (1)	D	740	376	64	306	1
Buster bar (1)	D	460	164	40	261	1
Dilly bar (1)	D	210	84	12	117	1
Milkshake, regular (1)	D	710	480	56	198	1
Malted milkshake, regular (1)	D	889	628	60	189	1

Food and Quantity	Starch Blocker Strategy Rating	Total Calories	Total Carbohydrate Calories	Total Protein Calories	Total Fat Calories	Fiber (g)
POPULAR FAST-FOOD RESTAURANTS *(continued)*						
Dairy Queen™:						
Freeze (1)	D	250	252	0	0	0
Hot Dog w/ chili (1)	D	320	92	52	180	2
Jack in the Box™:						
Breakfast Jack						
sandwich (1)	D	307	120	72	117	1
Hamburger (1)	D	276	120	48	108	1
Cheeseburger (1)	D	323	84	64	135	1
Jumbo Jack (1)	D	485	152	104	234	1
Bacon cheeseburger						
supreme (1)	D–	724	176	136	414	1
Swiss and baconburger						
(1)	F	643	124	132	387	1
Chicken supreme (1)	D	601	156	124	324	1
Moby Jack sandwich (1)	D	444	156	65	225	1
Taco, regular (1)	C–	191	64	32	99	1
Taco, supreme (1)	C–	288	84	48	153	1
Apple turnover (1)	D	410	180	16	216	1
Kentucky Fried Chicken™:						
Two-piece dinner,						
combination (1)	C–	661	192	132	342	1
Original Recipe:						
Center breast (1)	B	236	28	96	126	1
Side breast (1)	B	199	28	64	108	1
Drumstick (1)	B	117	12	48	63	1
Thigh (1)	B	257	28	72	162	1
Wing (1)	B	136	16	40	81	1
Extra-crispy recipe:						
Center breast (1)	B–	297	56	96	144	1
Side breast (1)	B–	286	56	68	162	1
Drumstick (1)	B–	155	20	52	81	1
Thigh (1)	B–	343	52	80	207	1
Wing (1)	B–	201	36	44	126	1
Mashed potatoes (.33 c)	B	60	48	8	9	1
Chicken gravy (.33 c)	C–	59	16	8	36	1
Dinner roll (1)	C	61	44	8	9	1
Kentucky nuggets (1)	B	46	8	12	27	1
Baked beans (.33 c)	B	177	68	24	81	1
Chicken Little						
sandwich (1)	B–	177	68	24	81	1

Food and Quantity	Starch Blocker Strategy Rating	Total Calories	Total Carbohydrate Calories	Total Protein Calories	Total Fat Calories	Fiber (g)
McDonalds™:						
Sandwiches:						
Big Mac (1)	D	560	172	100	288	1
McDLT sandwich (1)	D	580	144	104	378	1.4
Quarter Pounder (1)	D	410	136	92	189	1
Quarter Pounder w/ cheese (1)	D	520	140	116	261	1
Filet-O-Fish (1)	C+	440	152	56	234	1
French fries, small (1 srv)	D	220	104	16	108	1
Chicken McNuggets (6)	D	270	68	80	144	1
Sundaes:						
Hot fudge (1)	F	240	204	28	27	1
Strawberry (1)	D	210	196	24	9	1
Hot caramel (1)	F	270	236	28	27	1
Apple pie (1)	D	260	120	8	135	1
Egg McMuffin (1)	D	290	112	32.8	99	1
Hot cakes w/ butter & syrup (1)	D	410	296	32	81	1
Biscuit Sandwiches:						
Sausage & egg (1)	D	529	132	80	315	1
Bacon, egg, & cheese (1)	D–	440	132	72	234	1
Salads:						
Chef Salad (1)	A	230	32	84	117	2
Garden salad (1)	A	110	24	28	63	2
Chunky chicken salad (1)	A	140	20	92	27	2
Taco Bell™:						
Burritos:						
Bean (1)	C	357	216	52	90	8
Beef (1)	C–	403	156	88	153	2
Bean & beef (1)	C	381	184	68	126	5
Burrito supreme (1)	C	413	184	72	162	5
Fajita (1)	B	234	80	60	99	2
Tacos:						
Regular (1)	C	183	44	40	99	1
Taco bellgrande (1)	C–	355	72	72	207	2
Soft taco (1)	C	228	72	48	108	2

Food and Quantity	Starch Blocker Strategy Rating	Total Calories	Total Carbohydrate Calories	Total Protein Calories	Total Fat Calories	Fiber (g)
POPULAR FAST-FOOD RESTAURANTS *(continued)*						
Taco Bell™:						
Tostada, regular (1)	C	243	108	40	99	7
Mexican pizza (1)	C	575	160	84	432	5
Nachos:						
Nacho, regular (1)	D	356	152	28	171	1
Nacho bellgrande (1)	D	649	244	88	315	6
Pintos and cheese (1)	C–	190	76	36	81	7
Cinnamon Crispas (1)	D	259	108	12	135	1
Wendy's™:						
Hamburgers:						
Single, no toppings (1)	C	350	116	84	144	1
Double, no toppings (1)	D	560	128	164	306	1
Big Classic (1)	D	470	144	104	225	2
Cheeseburgers:						
Bacon cheeseburger (1)	F	460	92	116	252	1
Single, w/ all toppings (1)	D	548	128	120	297	2
Double, w/ all toppings (1)	D–	735	108	192	432	2
Baked potatoes:						
Plain (1)	B	250	208	24	9	5
Bacon and cheese (1)	C	570	228	76	270	5
Broccoli and cheese (1)	B–	500	216	52	225	5
Chili and cheese (1)	C–	510	252	88	180	8
Sour cream and chives (1)	C	460	212	28	216	5
Chili (1 c)	C	230	64	84	81	5
French fries, regular (1 srv)	C	306	152	16	135	1
Frosty dairy dessert (1 c)	D	354	212	28	117	0

Information extrapolated from various sources, including: United States Department of Agriculture; Whitney, Cataldo, and Rolfes, *Understanding Normal and Clinical Nutrition,* West Publishing Company, St. Paul MN, 1991; United States Surgeon General's Office; various private corporations, including: Arby's, Burger King, Dairy Queen, Jack in the Box, Kentucky Fried Chicken, McDonald's, Taco Bell, and Wendy's; UK Muscle, Internet site: http://www.uk-muscle.com/community/resources.calorielist.asp.

NINE

STARCH BLOCKER DIET MENU PLANS

Look at All This Food!

B ecause each of us is so different, we all must design our own, individualized starch blocker diets.

Yours should be based upon your own caloric needs, your fat-loss goals, your desired rate of fat loss, and your personal tastes and preferences. It should also take into account any possible food sensitivities that you may have.

The following menu plans were not devised with you, specifically, in mind, so you shouldn't slavishly follow any of them. However, one or more of them may reflect your own needs and tastes rather closely. If one does, try following it, or at least try patterning your own menu plans after it.

The first two sets of menu plans are for somewhat typical types of people. The first is for a 40-year-old, relatively sedentary, 150-pound female who wants to lose 18 pounds in about three months. The second is for a 35-year-old, 190-pound male who wants to lose 30 pounds in about five months. Because these people essentially reflect the norm, we offered seven-day sample weight loss menu plans for both of them, and one-day prototypes of weight maintenance plans.

At first glance, you'll wonder how anyone could ever lose weight while eating so much food. But when you notice how many starch calories are being neutralized, you'll understand how these menu plans result in weight loss.

In addition to the seven-day plans for these rather typical people, there are also one-day plans for a variety of people: athletes, completely sedentary people, people with allergies, vegetarians, fast-food eaters, gourmands, obese people, and people who are satisfied with their weight but who would enjoy eating somewhat more. The strategy fits a broad range of people!

In fact, it fits virtually anyone who would like to be healthier, slimmer, or more able to eat enjoyable foods without becoming overweight.

If one of these descriptions fits you, work out your own menu plan, and start the strategy today.

Note: In the menus, items marked by an asterisk (*) denote recipes included in Chapter Ten.

A SEVEN-DAY SAMPLE WEIGHT LOSS PLAN

Plus a One-day Sample Weight Maintenance Plan for a 40-year-old, 150-Pound, Lightly Active Female

Goal Weight: 132 pounds

Target Weight Loss: 18 pounds, or 1.5 pounds per week, for 12 weeks

Basal Metabolic Rate: 1,584

Job Activity Level: Light Physically Active (score of 1.2)

After-Work Activity Level: Household Helper (score of 0.01)

Exercise Activity Level: Sedentary (0 calories are burned per day through exercise. If she were to exercise, she would be able to increase her daily caloric needs, thus increasing her food amounts.)

Therefore, she needs 1,917 calories per day to maintain her body weight.

To lose 1.5 pounds per week, she must neutralize 5,250 starch calories per week, or 750 starch calories per day.

After taking starch blockers, her total caloric intake is reduced to 1,167 calories per day.

DAY 1:

FOOD	TOTAL CALORIES	NEUTRALIZED CALORIES	REMAINING CALORIES
BREAKFAST:			
Apple juice (1 cup)	106	2	104
Sourdough waffle, with 1 tsp whipped butter and 2 Tbsp maple syrup (an alternative could be 2 scrambled eggs prepared with 2 Tbsp milk and 1 tsp butter)	409	140	269
Totals:	**515**	**142**	**373**
SNACK:			
Whole wheat toast with 1 tsp butter	126	95	31
Hot chocolate (½ cup)	67	0	67
Totals:	**193**	**95**	**98**
LUNCH:			
Sliced cucumbers with garlic salt and pepper	30	6	24
Hot Turkey Sandwich* (an alternative could be an English Vegetarian Sandwich*, or a cold salmon salad)	204	53	151
Iced sun tea	0	0	0
Totals:	**234**	**59**	**175**
SNACK			
Whole Wheat Bread Sticks* (1)	60	38	22
Peppermint tea	0	0	0
Totals:	**60**	**38**	**22**

DINNER:

Italian Macaroni and Tomatoes* (an alternative could be Huntington Chicken*)			
Chicken*)	230	100	130
Fragrant Dilly Bread* (1 slice)	132	63	69
French Onion Soup*	227	86	141
Totals:	**589**	**249**	**340**

DESSERT:

Angel Cake* (1 slice)	168	30	138
Total:	**168**	**30**	**138**
DAILY TOTALS:	**1,759**	**613**	**1,146**

DAY 2:

FOOD	TOTAL CALORIES	NEUTRALIZED CALORIES	REMAINING CALORIES
BREAKFAST:			
Honeydew melon (⅓)	148	0	148
2 poached or boiled eggs with 1 slice of whole wheat toast and 1 tsp butter	286	98	188
Tea or coffee with milk	10	0	10
Totals:	**444**	**98**	**346**
SNACK:			
Tomato juice (1 cup)	50	0	50
Chex™ mix (½ cup)	45	34	11
Totals:	**95**	**34**	**61**

LUNCH:

Food	Total	Neutralized	Remaining
English Vegetarian Sandwich* (an alternative could be Chicken and Rice Casserole*)	198	53	145
Potato chips (10)	110	40	70
Cucumber Slaw*	28	4	24
2% milk (½ cup)	60	0	60
Totals:	**396**	**97**	**299**

SNACK:

Food	Total	Neutralized	Remaining
Popcorn (1 cup)	65	49	16
Total:	**65**	**49**	**16**

DINNER:

Food	Total	Neutralized	Remaining
Cajun Cod and Rice* (an alternative could be Escalloped Oysters*)	221	76	145
Asparagus (6–8 spears)	20	6	14
Heavenly Biscuit* (1)	111	63	48
Lyonnaise Potatoes*	149	18	131
Red wine (1 glass)	74	0	74
Totals:	**575**	**163**	**412**
DAILY TOTALS:	**1,575**	**441**	**1,134**

DAY 3:

FOOD	TOTAL CALORIES	NEUTRALIZED CALORIES	REMAINING CALORIES
BREAKFAST:			
Grapefruit (½) or apple (½)	45	2	43
Cornflakes (1 cup) with 1 tsp sugar and ½ cup 2% milk (an alternative could be 1 poached egg on 1 piece of toast)	177	84	93

English muffin with 1 tsp butter	132	42	90
Totals:	**354**	**128**	**226**

SNACK:

Frozen banana, dipped in chocolate	140	18	122
Total:	**140**	**18**	**122**

LUNCH:

Western Chili* (an alternative could be a Hot Turkey Sandwich*)	291	141	150
Saltine crackers (6)	105	79	26
Crunchy Apple Salad*	158	8	150
Totals:	**554**	**228**	**326**

SNACK:

Beef noodle soup (1 cup)	70	0	70
4 crackers	70	53	17
Totals:	**140**	**53**	**87**

DINNER:

Huntington Chicken* (an alternative could be a Salmon Loaf*)	242	76	166
Baked potato with 2 Tbsp yogurt and chopped chives	136	100	36
Honey Minted Carrots*	68	5	63
Totals:	**446**	**181**	**265**

DESSERT:

Angel food cake (1 piece)	143	29	114
Total:	**143**	**29**	**114**
DAILY TOTALS:	**1,777**	**637**	**1,140**

DAY 4:

FOOD	TOTAL CALORIES	NEUTRALIZED CALORIES	REMAINING CALORIES
BREAKFAST:			
Orange juice (½ cup)	56	0	56
1 scrambled egg, prepared with 1 Tbsp milk and ½ tsp butter	110	0	110
Whole wheat toast with 1 tsp whipped butter (1 slice)	126	95	31
Totals:	**292**	**95**	**197**
SNACK:			
Toasted bagel (½) with tomato and slice of cheese	240	80	160
Herb tea	0	0	0
Totals:	**240**	**80**	**160**
LUNCH:			
½ serving of Lazy Day Spaghetti* (an alternative could be ½ Hot Crab Sandwich*)	49	5	44
Sautéed zucchini (1 cup)	40	4	36
Pear (1)	100	8	92
Totals:	**240**	**71**	**169**
SNACK:			
Celery with 2 Tbsp all-natural (no additives) peanut butter	91	9	82
Whole Wheat Bread Sticks* (2)	120	76	44
Cold chocolate milk (½ cup)	67	0	67
Totals:	**278**	**85**	**193**

DINNER:

Food	Total Calories	Neutralized Calories	Remaining Calories
Barbecued top sirloin (4 oz) (an alternative could be Baked Chicken Stew*, or grilled halibut)	320	0	320
Baked potato with 2 Tbsp yogurt and chopped chives	136	100	36
Hearty Bean and Carrot Salad*	127	45	82
Totals:	**583**	**145**	**438**
DAILY TOTALS:	**1,582**	**422**	**1,160**

DAY 5:

FOOD	TOTAL CALORIES	NEUTRALIZED CALORIES	REMAINING CALORIES
BREAKFAST:			
Pineapple chunks with nutmeg and crushed almonds (½ cup)	60	1	59
½ cup rice and raisins, with 2 tsp brown sugar and ¼ cup skim milk	238	90	148
Whole wheat toast, 1 tsp honey (1 slice)	131	98	33
Totals:	**429**	**189**	**240**
SNACK:			
Cornbread* (1 piece)	118	49	69
Total:	**118**	**49**	**69**
LUNCH:			
Egg Salad Sandwich* (an alternative could be a Hot Turkey Sandwich*)	372	173	199

Boston's Best Baked Beans*	251	132	119
Tomato, with garlic and pepper (1)	30	0	30
Totals:	**653**	**305**	**348**

SNACK:

Yogurt (1 cup)	120	0	120
Total:	**120**	**0**	**120**

DINNER:

Split pea soup*	203	100	103
Grilled ocean perch (3 oz), with Bermuda onions (an alternative could be Italian Macroni and Tomatoes*)	120	0	120
Boiled new potatoes*	200	150	50
Whole Wheat Bread Sticks* (2)	120	76	44
Succotash*	99	74	25
Totals:	**742**	**400**	**342**
DAILY TOTALS:	**2,062**	**943**	**1,119**

DAY 6:

FOOD	**TOTAL CALORIES**	**NEUTRALIZED CALORIES**	**REMAINING CALORIES**
BREAKFAST:			
All-Bran cereal (1 cup), with 1 sliced banana, 2 tsp brown sugar, and ½ cup skim milk	255	160	95
Whole wheat toast, 1 tsp butter (1 slice)	126	95	31
Totals:	**381**	**255**	**126**

SNACK:

Banana Nut Bread* (1 slice)	150	43	107
Earl Grey tea	0	0	0
Totals:	**150**	**43**	**107**

LUNCH:

French Toasted Sandwich* (an alternative could be Veal Stew with Parsley Dumplings*)	360	165	195
Tossed green salad	32	0	32
Sliced peach with honey and cinnamon	60	2	58
Totals:	**452**	**167**	**285**

SNACK:

Crackers with all-natural (no additives) peanut butter (4)	150	90	60
Whole wheat cracker	17	12	15
Milk (½ cup 1%)	51	0	51
Totals:	**218**	**102**	**116**

DINNER:

Tahitian Chicken* (an alternative could be Stuffed Cube Steaks*)	330	52	8
Steamed rice (white or brown)	200	150	50
Beijing Pea Pod Salad*	42	0	42
Baked Apple	169	8	161
Totals:	**741**	**210**	**531**
DAILY TOTALS:	**1,942**	**777**	**1,165**

DAY 7:

FOOD	TOTAL CALORIES	NEUTRALIZED CALORIES	REMAINING CALORIES
SUNDAY BRUNCH:			
Melon ball compote	23	0	23
Scrambled eggs (2) with mushrooms	240	0	240
Potato Kugel*	277	170	107
Popover* with 1 tsp whipped butter	70	38	32
Totals:	**610**	**208**	**402**
SUPPER:			
Turkey with dressing (4 oz)	361	100	261
Mashed potatoes with garlic butter (1 cup)	360	270	90
Turkey gravy (½ cup)	30	0	30
Green beans (1 cup)	30	0	30
Dinner roll with 1 tsp whipped butter	123	90	33
Totals:	**904**	**460**	**444**
DESSERT:			
Pumpkin pie	316	19	297
Total:	**316**	**19**	**297**
DAILY TOTALS:	**1,830**	**687**	**1,143**

ONE-DAY SAMPLE WEIGHT MAINTENANCE PLAN FOR A 40-YEAR-OLD, FORMERLY 150-POUND, LIGHTLY ACTIVE FEMALE—NOW 132 POUNDS

Goal Weight: maintain present weight of 132 pounds

Target Weight Loss: none

Basal Metabolic Rate: 1,394

Job Activity Level: Light Physically Active (score of 1.2)

After-Work Activity Level: Household Helper (score of 0.01)

Exercise Activity Level: Sedentary (0 calories are burned per day through exercise. If she were to exercise, she would be able to increase her daily caloric needs, thus increasing her food amounts.)

Therefore, she needs 1,686 calories per day to maintain her body weight.

FOOD	TOTAL CALORIES	NEUTRALIZED CALORIES	REMAINING CALORIES
BREAKFAST:			
Potato Pancakes* (2)	190	96	94
Sourdough waffle, with 1 tsp whipped butter and 2 Tbsp syrup	409	140	269
Skim milk (1 small glass)	77	0	77
Totals:	**676**	**236**	**440**
SNACK:			
Heavenly Biscuit* (1)	111	63	48
Frozen banana, dipped in chocolate	140	18	122
Totals:	**251**	**81**	**170**
LUNCH:			
Tostada with refried beans (1)	212	150	62
Beef taco on corn tortilla (1)	207	52	155

Coleslaw (½ cup)	89	8	81
Tortilla chips (1 oz)	70	10	60
Totals:	**578**	**220**	**358**

SNACK:

Apple (½)	45	9	36
Crackers with all-natural (no additives) peanut butter (4)	150	90	60
Totals:	**195**	**99**	**96**

DINNER:

Roasted Butternut Squash Soup*	112	8	104
Barbecued chicken (½ breast and 1 drumstick) (an alternative could be Tamale Pie*, or Crab Louis)	218	0	218
Mashed potatoes and gravy	340	188	152
Hearty Bean and Carrot Salad*	127	45	82
Garden salad with low-fat dressing	50	10	40
Totals:	**847**	**251**	**596**
DAILY TOTALS:	**2,547**	**887**	**1,660**

A SEVEN-DAY SAMPLE WEIGHT LOSS PLAN

Plus a One-day Sample Weight Maintenance Plan for a 35-year-old, 190-Pound, Moderately Active Male

Goal Weight: 160 pounds

Target Weight Loss: 30 pounds, or 1.5 pounds per week, for 20 weeks

Basal Metabolic Rate: 2,212

Job Activity Level: Moderately Active Job (score of 1.3)

After-Work Activity Level: Couch Potato (score of 0.00)

Exercise Activity Level: Light (Averages 15 minutes a day, burning an average of 163 calories per day by playing basketball for about an hour, twice a week, for a total of 1,141 calories per week.)

Therefore, he needs 3,039 calories per day to maintain his body weight.

To lose 1.5 pounds per week, he must neutralize 5,250 starch calories per week, or 750 starch calories per day.

After taking starch blockers, his total caloric intake is reduced to 2,289 calories per day.

7-DAY MENU PLANS

DAY 1:

FOOD	TOTAL CALORIES	NEUTRALIZED CALORIES	REMAINING CALORIES
BREAKFAST:			
Cantaloupe (½)	90	6	84
2 egg omelette with ½ cup mushrooms	200	0	200
Whole wheat toast (1 slice) with 1 tsp butter	126	95	31

Fresh orange juice (1½ cups)	160	8	152
Coffee or tea	0	0	0
Totals:	**576**	**109**	**467**

SNACK:

Sliced banana with maple syrup and cashews	143	20	123
Pretzels (18 pieces)	110	69	41
Total:	**253**	**89**	**164**

LUNCH:

Vegetable Soup*	169	92	77
Hot Crab Sandwich* (an alternative could be Lazy Day Spaghetti*)	139	53	86
Oven baked french fries (20)	340	160	180
Garden salad with low-fat dressing	50	10	40
Totals:	**698**	**315**	**383**

SNACK:

English muffin with ½ tsp butter	115	42	73
Skim milk (1 glass)	90	0	90
Totals:	**205**	**42**	**163**

DINNER:

Barbecued chicken (2 pieces) (an alternative could be a broiled 4 oz New York steak)	378	0	378
Scalloped Potatoes Au Gratin*	257	97	160
Corn on the cob (1)	100	63	37
Cornbread* (1 piece)	118	49	69
Pear (1)	100	24	76
Microbrew beer (1 pint)	292	0	292
Totals:	**1,245**	**233**	**1,012**

DESSERT:

Orange Almond Biscotti* (2)	130	30	100
Total:	**130**	**30**	**100**
DAILY TOTALS:	**3,107**	**818**	**2,289**

DAY 2:

FOOD	TOTAL CALORIES	NEUTRALIZED CALORIES	REMAINING CALORIES
BREAKFAST:			
Fresh orange juice (1½ cups)	160	8	152
Sourdough pancakes (4), with 2 tsp butter and 3 Tbsp syrup	368	140	228
Bacon (2 slices)	90	0	90
Whole milk (1 cup)	150	0	150
Totals:	**768**	**148**	**620**
SNACK:			
Blueberry Cornmeal Muffin* (1)	321	43	278
Coffee or mint tea	0	0	0
Totals:	**321**	**43**	**278**
LUNCH:			
McDonald's Chicken McGrill Sandwich	410	100	310
Small french fries	220	105	115
Chocolate milkshake (10 oz)	320	0	320
Totals:	**950**	**205**	**745**
SNACK:			
Apple (1)	90	18	72
Whole Wheat Bread Sticks* (2)	120	72	48

Food	TOTAL CALORIES	NEUTRALIZED CALORIES	REMAINING CALORIES
Coffee	0	0	0
Total:	**210**	**90**	**120**
DINNER:			
Broiled New York steak (4 oz) (an alternative could be Baked Chicken Stew*)	320	0	320
Dinner rolls (2), with 2 tsp whipped butter	246	180	66
Mashed potatoes with garlic butter (1 cup)	360	270	90
Corn on the cob (1)	100	63	37
Totals:	**1,026**	**513**	**513**
DAILY TOTALS:	**3,275**	**999**	**2,276**

DAY 3:

FOOD	TOTAL CALORIES	NEUTRALIZED CALORIES	REMAINING CALORIES
BREAKFAST:			
Whole milk (1 cup)	150	0	150
Potato Pancakes* (2)	190	96	94
Eggs fried in butter (2)	180	0	180
Coffee	0	0	0
Totals:	**520**	**96**	**424**
SNACK:			
Tomato soup (1 cup)	50	0	50
Jalapeño Cornbread* (1 piece)	318	83	235
Totals:	**368**	**83**	**285**

LUNCH:

Food			
Barley Soup* (an alternative could be Roasted Butternut Squash Soup*)	331	217	114
Spaghetti Pie*	284	115	169
Garden salad with low-fat dressing	50	10	40
Totals:	**665**	**342**	**323**

SNACK:

Food			
Popcorn (1 cup)	65	49	16
Diet Pepsi on ice (1 glass)	0	0	0
Totals:	**65**	**49**	**16**

DINNER:

Food			
Imported beer (12 oz)	146	0	146
Prime beef, roasted with pearl onions (6 oz) (an alternative could be Seafood Fettuccine Vin Blanc*)	765	15	750
Scalloped Potatoes Au Gratin*	257	97	160
Dinner roll with 1 tsp butter	123	90	33
Split Pea Soup*	203	100	103
Asparagus (6–8 spears)	20	6	14
Totals:	**1,514**	**308**	**1,206**
DAILY TOTALS:	**3,132**	**878**	**2,254**

DAY 4:

FOOD	TOTAL CALORIES	NEUTRALIZED CALORIES	REMAINING CALORIES
BREAKFAST:			
Cinnamon Crunch Bread* (1 slice)	211	92	119
Grapefruit (1)	45	8	37

Whole wheat toast with 1 tsp butter (1 slice)	126	95	31
Whole milk (½ cup)	75	0	75
Totals:	**457**	**195**	**262**

SNACK:

Quick Chicken Noodle Soup*	143	77	66
Total:	**143**	**77**	**66**

LUNCH:

Shrimp Chow Mein* (an alternative could be Ginger Rice*)	208	93	115
Steamed rice (2 cups)	400	300	100
Egg rolls (2)	308	30	278
Hot green tea	0	0	0
Totals:	**916**	**423**	**493**

SNACK:

Popcorn (1 cup)	65	49	16
Fresh orange juice (1 cup)	60	1	59
Totals:	**125**	**50**	**75**

DINNER:

Pinot Gris wine (1 glass)	74	0	74
Appetizer of smoked oysters (6)	135	0	135
Seafood Fettuccini Vin Blanc* (an alternative could be 6 oz prime beef, roasted with pearl onions)	781	59	722
Broccoli with white sauce	221	56	165
Yam Fluff*	177	90	87
Garden salad with low-fat vinaigrette dressing	50	10	40
Totals:	**1,438**	**215**	**1,223**

DESSERT:

Bread Pudding*	209	41	168
Totals:	**209**	**41**	**168**
DAILY TOTALS:	**3,288**	**1,001**	**2,287**

DAY 5:

FOOD	TOTAL CALORIES	NEUTRALIZED CALORIES	REMAINING CALORIES
BREAKFAST:			
Oatmeal (2 cups) with 1 tsp honey and ¼ cup skim milk	175	80	95
Banana Nut Bread* (1 slice)	150	43	107
Cantaloupe (¼)	45	1	44
Totals:	**370**	**124**	**246**
SNACK:			
Anadama Bread* (1 slice)	116	68	48
Chex™ mix (½ cup)	45	34	11
Apple (1)	90	18	72
Totals:	**251**	**120**	**131**
LUNCH:			
Baked Chicken Stew* (an alternative could be Chicken with Chanterelle Cream Sauce and Fettuccine*)	419	83	336
Chinese Fried Rice*	205	100	105
Croque Monsieur*	724	88	636
Whole milk (1 cup)	150	0	150
Totals:	**1,498**	**271**	**1,227**

SNACK:

Food			
Hearty Bean and Carrot Salad*	127	45	82
Doughnut (1 cake type, plain)	210	52	158
Total:	**337**	**97**	**240**

DINNER:

Food			
Swiss steak (an alternative could be Tahitian Chicken*, or pan-fried halibut)	281	7	274
Stuffed potato	124	93	31
Vegetable Soup*	169	92	77
Dinner rolls (2) with 1 tsp whipped butter	213	180	33
Totals:	**787**	**372**	**415**
DAILY TOTALS:	**3,243**	**984**	**2,259**

DAY 6:

FOOD	**TOTAL CALORIES**	**NEUTRALIZED CALORIES**	**REMAINING CALORIES**
BREAKFAST:			
2 egg omelette	220	0	220
Corn grits (½ cup) with 1 tsp butter, sugar, 2 Tbsp milk	153	115	38
Prune juice (1 cup), or orange juice	187	18	169
Sourdough waffle, with 1 tsp whipped butter and 2 Tbsp syrup	409	140	269
Totals:	**969**	**273**	**696**

SNACK:

Whole milk (1 cup)	150	0	150
Whole Wheat Bread Sticks* (2)	120	76	44
Totals:	**270**	**76**	**194**

LUNCH:

Turkey sandwich (an alternative could be a ham or roast beef sandwich)	259	56	203
Macaroni salad (1 cup)	297	148	149
Blueberry Cornmeal Muffin*	231	43	188
Totals:	**787**	**247**	**540**

SNACK:

Orange (1)	60	1	59
Tortilla chips (1 oz)	150	57	93
Totals:	**210**	**58**	**152**

DINNER:

Broiled Salmon (3 oz) (an alternative could be Chicken and Rice Casserole*)	183	0	183
Grilled Polenta with Piperade Basquaise*	325	58	267
Steamed rice (white or brown, 1 cup)	200	150	50
Totals:	**708**	**208**	**500**

DESSERT:

Cherry cobbler (1 piece)	199	46	153
Total:	**199**	**46**	**153**
DAILY TOTALS:	**3,143**	**908**	**2,235**

DAY 7:

FOOD	TOTAL CALORIES	NEUTRALIZED CALORIES	REMAINING CALORIES
BREAKFAST:			
Corn Chex™ with milk (1 cup each)	261	83	178
2 poached eggs on 2 pieces of toast	290	105	185
Sliced banana with 2 Tbsp honey-yogurt topping, 1 tsp crushed cashews	143	20	123
Fresh orange juice (1½ cups)	160	8	152
Totals:	**854**	**216**	**638**
SNACK:			
Pretzels (18)	110	69	41
Apple juice (1½ cups)	160	6	154
Totals:	**270**	**75**	**195**
LUNCH:			
Tuna salad sandwich (an alternative could be a French Toasted Sandwich*)	309	142	167
Potato chips (10)	110	40	70
Chicken noodle soup	75	30	45
Milk (1 cup)	150	0	150
Hearty Bean and Carrot Salad*	127	45	82
Totals:	**771**	**257**	**514**

SNACK:

Whole wheat toast, with 1 tsp butter	126	95	31
Hot chocolate (½ cup)	67	0	67
Totals:	**193**	**95**	**98**

DINNER:

Bean burrito (1)	322	242	80
Beef taco	207	52	155
Spanish Rice	264	75	189
Refried beans (½ cup)	135	63	72
Green bean salad	48	1	47
Totals:	**976**	**433**	**543**

DESSERT:

Orange Almond Biscotti* (2)	130	30	100
Milk (1 cup)	150	0	150
Decaf coffee or herb tea	0	0	0
Totals:	**280**	**30**	**250**
DAILY TOTALS:	**3,344**	**1,106**	**2,238**

ONE-DAY SAMPLE WEIGHT MAINTENANCE PLAN FOR A 35-YEAR-OLD, FORMERLY 190-POUND, MODERATELY ACTIVE MALE—NOW 160 POUNDS

Goal Weight: maintain present weight of 160 pounds

Target Weight Loss: none

Basal Metabolic Rate: 1,853

Job Activity Level: Moderately Active Job (score of 1.3)

After-Work Activity Level: Couch Potato (score of 0.00)

Exercise Activity Level: Light (Averages 15 minutes a day, burning an average of 163 calories per day by playing basketball for about an hour, twice a week, for a total of 1,141 calories per week.)

Therefore, he needs 2,571 calories per day to maintain his body weight.

FOOD	TOTAL CALORIES	NEUTRALIZED CALORIES	REMAINING CALORIES
BREAKFAST:			
Biscuits (2) and gravy (⅓ cup)	524	188	336
Cantaloupe (½)	90	6	84
2 poached eggs on 2 pieces of toast	290	105	185
Fresh orange juice (1 cup)	60	1	59
Totals:	**964**	**300**	**664**
SNACK:			
Sliced banana with 2 Tbsp honey-yogurt topping, and 1 tsp crushed cashews	143	20	123
Graham crackers (2)	60	23	37
Coffee or mint tea	0	0	0
Totals:	**203**	**43**	**160**

LUNCH:

Lasagna, w/ meat (1 serving) (an alternative could be Grilled Polenta with Piperade Basquaise*)	398	150	248
Italian bread (2 slices)	166	125	41
Garden salad with low-fat dressing	50	10	40
Minestrone soup	227	86	141
Totals:	**841**	**371**	**470**

SNACK:

Chocolate PowerBar	225	84	141
Fresh orange juice (1½ cups)	160	8	152
Totals:	**385**	**92**	**293**

DINNER:

Burgundy wine (1 glass)	74	0	74
Broiled New York steak (4 oz) (an alternative could be Chicken with Chanterelle Cream Sauce and Fettuccine*, or a grilled tuna fillet)	320	0	320
Mashed potatoes and gravy	340	188	152
Cauliflower with cheese sauce	174	12	162
Hearty Bean and Carrot Salad*	127	45	82
Dinner roll	50	37	13
Corn on the cob (1)	84	37	47
Totals:	**1,169**	**319**	**850**

DESSERT:

Chocolate brownie	194	60	134
Decaf coffee or herb tea	0	0	0
Totals:	**194**	**60**	**134**
DAILY TOTALS:	**3,756**	**1,185**	**2,571**

SAMPLE ONE-DAY WEIGHT MANAGEMENT MENU PLANS FOR VARIOUS TYPES OF PEOPLE

Sample Weight Loss Menu for 35-year-old, 155-Pound Very Active, Athletic Female

Goal Weight: 145 pounds

Target Weight Loss: 10 pounds, or 2 pounds per week, for 5 weeks

Basal Metabolic Rate: 1,654

Job Activity Level: Light Physically Active (score of 1.2)

After-Work Activity Level: Go-getter (score of 0.02)

Exercise Activity Level: Very active (2 hours a day, burning 1,236 calories per day on a stair machine)

Therefore, she needs 3,254 calories per day to maintain her body weight.

To lose 2 pounds per week, she must neutralize 7,000 starch calories per week, or 1,000 starch calories per day.

After taking starch blockers, her total caloric intake is reduced to 2,254 calories per day.

FOOD	TOTAL CALORIES	NEUTRALIZED CALORIES	REMAINING CALORIES
BREAKFAST:			
Coffee or tea, with milk	10	0	10
2 poached eggs on 2 pieces of toast (an alternative could be waffles, or cereal with milk)	290	105	185
Potato Pancake* (1)	95	48	47
Sliced orange (½)	30	1	29
Totals:	**425**	**154**	**271**
SNACK:			
Cinnamon Crunch Bread* (1 slice)	211	92	119

Whole milk (1 cup)	150	0	150
Totals:	**361**	**92**	**269**

LUNCH:

Seafood Fettuccine Vin Blanc* (an alternative could be Croque Monsieur*)	781	59	722
Sliced banana with 2 Tbsp honey-yogurt topping, and 1 tsp crushed cashews	143	20	123
Totals:	**924**	**79**	**845**

SNACK:

Toasted bagel, both halves, with all-fruit jelly	210	80	130
Apple juice (½ glass)	116	5	111
Totals:	**326**	**85**	**241**

DINNER:

Huntington Chicken* (an alternative could be Quick Shrimp and Rice*)	242	76	166
Mashed potatoes with garlic butter (1 cup)	360	270	90
Garden salad with low-fat dressing	50	10	40
Steamed artichoke (1)	60	36	24
Dinner roll with 1 tsp butter	123	90	33
Totals:	**835**	**482**	**353**

DESSERT:

Raisin rice pudding	295	38	257
Total:	**295**	**38**	**257**
DAILY TOTALS:	**3,166**	**930**	**2,236**

SAMPLE WEIGHT LOSS MENU FOR A 35-YEAR-OLD, 185-POUND VERY ACTIVE, ATHLETIC MALE

Goal Weight: 171 pounds

Target Weight Loss: 14 pounds, or 2 pounds per week, for 7 weeks

Basal Metabolic Rate: 2,153

Job Activity Level: Light Physically Active (score of 1.2)

After-Work Activity Level: Go-getter (score of 0.02)

Exercise Activity Level: Very active (2 hours a day, burning 1,236 calories per day)

Therefore, he needs 3,863 calories per day to maintain his body weight.

To lose 2 pounds per week, he must neutralize 7,000 starch calories per week, or 1,000 starch calories per day.

After taking starch blockers, his total caloric intake is reduced to 2,863 calories per day.

FOOD	TOTAL CALORIES	NEUTRALIZED CALORIES	REMAINING CALORIES
BREAKFAST:			
Bacon (3 slices)	135	0	135
Cantaloupe (½)	90	6	84
2 boiled eggs and 2 pieces of toast	290	105	185
Totals:	**515**	**111**	**404**
SNACK:			
Chocolate PowerBar	225	84	141
Crackers with all-natural (no additives) peanut butter (4)	150	90	60
Totals:	**375**	**174**	**201**

LUNCH:

Grilled cheese sandwich (an alternative could be hot beef stew)	399	98	301
Cinnamon Crunch Bread* (1 slice)	211	92	119
Tomato soup with milk (1 cup)	161	0	161
Potato chips (20)	220	80	140
Chicken salad	104	0	104
Milk (2 cups)	300	0	300
Totals:	**1,395**	**270**	**1,125**

SNACK:

Anadama Bread* (1 slice)	116	68	48
Chex™ mix (½ cup)	45	34	11
Apple (1)	90	18	72
Totals:	**251**	**120**	**131**

DINNER:

Deep Dish Pizza* (an alternative could be Creamed Chicken and Asparagus*, or tuna casserole)	265	95	170
Stuffed Green Pepper*	244	75	169
French bread (2 slices) with 2 Tbsp garlic butter	400	100	300
Tossed green salad	32	0	32
Totals:	**941**	**270**	**671**

DESSERT:

Chocolate Hazelnut Shortcake with White Chocolate Cream and Berries*	364	57	307
Total:	**364**	**57**	**307**
DAILY TOTALS:	**3,841**	**1,002**	**2,839**

SAMPLE WEIGHT LOSS MENU FOR A 54-YEAR-OLD, 160-POUND SEDENTARY FEMALE

Goal Weight: 135 pounds

Target Weight Loss: 25 pounds, or 1.5 pounds per week, for 17 weeks

Basal Metabolic Rate: 1,637

Job Activity Level: Sedentary (score of 1.1)

After-Work Activity Level: Couch Potato (score of 0.00)

Exercise Activity Level: Sedentary (0 calories are burned per day through exercise. If she were to exercise, she would be able to increase her daily caloric needs, thus increasing her food amounts.)

Therefore, she needs 1,801 calories per day to maintain her body weight.

To lose 1.5 pounds per week, she must neutralize 5,250 starch calories per week, or 750 starch calories per day.

After taking starch blockers, her total caloric intake is reduced to 1,051 calories per day.

FOOD	TOTAL CALORIES	NEUTRALIZED CALORIES	REMAINING CALORIES
BREAKFAST:			
Fresh pineapple chunks (½ cup)	40	3	37
Whole wheat toast (1 slice) with 1 tsp butter	126	95	31
Coffee or tea	0	0	0
Totals:	**166**	**98**	**68**
SNACK:			
Vanilla wafers (8)	148	87	61
Totals:	**148**	**87**	**61**

LUNCH:

All-natural (no additives) peanut butter and jam sandwich (an alternative could be a hamburger)	347	124	223
Potato chips (10)	110	40	70
Quick Chicken Noodle Soup*	143	77	66
Diet Pepsi on ice with a slice of lemon	1	0	1
Totals:	**601**	**241**	**360**

SNACK:

Watermelon (2 cups diced)	90	3	87
Graham crackers (2)	60	23	37
Totals:	**150**	**26**	**124**

DINNER:

Macaroni and Cheese* (an alternative could be Shrimp Chow Mein*)	207	81	126
French bread (1 slice) with ½ Tbsp butter	150	18	132
Good Old-Fashioned Potato Soup*	175	90	85
Garden salad with low-fat dressing	50	10	40
Milk (½ cup 1%)	51	0	51
Totals:	**633**	**199**	**434**
DAILY TOTALS:	**1,698**	**651**	**1,047**

SAMPLE WEIGHT LOSS MENU FOR A 52-YEAR-OLD, 145-POUND FEMALE WITH FOOD ALLERGIES (TO WHEAT, DAIRY PRODUCTS, AND EGGS)

Goal Weight: 125 pounds

Target Weight Loss: 20 pounds, or 1 pound per week, for 20 weeks

Basal Metabolic Rate: 1,499

Job Activity Level: Moderately Active (score of 1.3)

After-Work Activity Level: Household Helper (score of 0.01)

Exercise Activity Level: None

Therefore, she needs 1,964 calories per day to maintain her body weight.

To lose 1 pound per week, she must neutralize 3,500 starch calories per week, or about 500 starch calories per day.

After taking starch blockers, her total caloric intake is reduced to 1,464 calories per day.

FOOD	TOTAL CALORIES	NEUTRALIZED CALORIES	REMAINING CALORIES
BREAKFAST:			
Fruit salad with sweetened soy yogurt (1 cup), and ½ cup cashews or walnuts	330	50	280
Tea with ½ tsp honey	20	0	20
Totals:	**350**	**50**	**300**
SNACK:			
Rice cake (1) with 1 Tbsp nut butter and 1 tsp all-fruit jam	250	70	180
Total:	**250**	**70**	**180**
LUNCH:			
Tuna salad (large) with 1 can of solid albacore in water, and 1 Tbsp low-fat vinaigrette dressing.			

Salad contains lettuce, tomato, zucchini, cucumber, carrots, and sprouts (an alternative could be Smoked Salmon Hash*)	365	50	315
Total:	**365**	**50**	**315**
SNACK:			
Apple (1)	90	18	72
Tea with ½ tsp honey	20	0	20
Totals:	**110**	**18**	**92**
DINNER:			
Cocktail (2 oz vodka with orange juice)	160	0	160
Grilled chicken (2 skinless breasts) with lemon, garlic, and tamari (an alternative could be Dutch Cabbage Rolls*)	161	0	161
Corn on the cob (1) or serving of another starchy vegetable, with ½ tsp soy butter or olive oil	120	63	57
Asparagus (6–8 spears)	20	6	14
Rice bread with ½ tsp soy butter	100	75	25
Green salad with 1 Tbsp low-fat dressing	50	10	40
Baked potato with 1 tsp soy butter	165	112	53
Totals:	**776**	**266**	**510**
DESSERT:			
Ice cream with chocolate sauce (½ cup)	65	0	65
Total:	**65**	**0**	**65**
DAILY TOTALS:	**1,916**	**454**	**1,462**

SAMPLE WEIGHT LOSS MENU FOR A 25-YEAR-OLD, 130-POUND FEMALE VEGETARIAN

Goal Weight: 120 pounds

Target Weight Loss: 10 pounds, or 1.5 pounds per week, for 7 weeks

Basal Metabolic Rate: 1,416

Job Activity Level: Light Physically Active (score of 1.2)

After-Work Activity Level: Go-getter (score of 0.02)

Exercise Activity Level: Very Active (1 hour per day fast jogging)

Therefore, she needs 2,358 calories per day to maintain her body weight.

To lose 1.5 pounds per week, she must neutralize 5,250 starch calories per week, or about 750 starch calories per day.

After taking starch blockers, her total caloric intake is reduced to 1,608 calories per day.

FOOD	TOTAL CALORIES	NEUTRALIZED CALORIES	REMAINING CALORIES
BREAKFAST:			
Bagel with 1 Tbsp tofu cream cheese	190	72	118
Sliced banana with 2 Tbsp honey-yogurt topping, 1 tsp crushed cashews	143	20	123
Fresh orange juice (1 cup)	60	1	59
Totals:	**393**	**93**	**300**
SNACK:			
Anadama Bread* (1 slice)	116	68	48
Soy milk (½ cup)	65	9	56
Total:	**181**	**77**	**104**

LUNCH:

All-natural (no additives) peanut butter and jam sandwich (an alternative could be a grilled cheese sandwich)	347	124	223
Red Kidney Bean Salad*	405	199	206
Apple juice (1 cup)	106	2	104
Totals:	**858**	**325**	**533**

SNACK:

Yogurt (1 cup)	120	0	120
Fresh pineapple chunks (½ cup)	40	3	37
Graham cracker (1)	30	12	19
Totals:	**190**	**15**	**176**

DINNER:

Western Chili* (no meat added) (an alternative could be two servings of the Vegetable Burger Bake*)	220	141	79
Cornbread*	118	49	69
Cooked okra (½ cup)	25	12	13
Garden salad with low-fat dressing	50	10	40
Soy milk (1 cup)	130	18	112
Totals:	**543**	**230**	**313**

DESSERT:

Tofutti Frutti ice cream bar	180	20	160
Tea with ½ tsp honey	20	0	20
Totals:	**200**	**20**	**180**
DAILY TOTALS:	**2,366**	**760**	**1,606**

SAMPLE WEIGHT LOSS MENU FOR A 36-YEAR-OLD, 180-POUND MALE FAST-FOOD EATER

Goal Weight: 152 pounds

Target Weight Loss: 28 pounds, or 2 pounds per week, for 14 weeks

Basal Metabolic Rate: 2,095

Job Activity Level: Very Active (score of 1.4)

After-Work Activity Level: Household Helper (score of 0.01)

Exercise Activity Level: Moderately Active (30 minutes per day medium weight training)

Therefore, he needs 3,200 calories per day to maintain his body weight.

To lose 2 pounds per week, he must neutralize 7,000 starch calories per week, or about 1,000 starch calories per day.

After taking starch blockers, his total caloric intake is reduced to 2,200 calories per day.

FOOD	TOTAL CALORIES	NEUTRALIZED CALORIES	REMAINING CALORIES
BREAKFAST:			
McDonald's Egg McMuffin	300	60	240
McDonald's hash browns (2)	260	98	162
Orange juice (16 oz)	180	6	174
Totals:	**740**	**164**	**576**
SNACK:			
Vending machine cheese crackers (10)	50	19	31
7-Eleven's blueberry muffin (1)	135	75	60
Coffee or tea	0	0	0
Totals:	**185**	**94**	**91**

LUNCH:

Pizza Hut hand-tossed Veggie Lovers pizza (2 slices)	440	84	356
Pizza Hut garlic bread (1 slice)	150	48	102
Pizza Hut chef salad	150	8	142
Diet Coca-Cola (1 glass with ice)	0	0	0
Totals:	**740**	**140**	**600**

SNACK:

Wendy's sour cream and chives potato with butter	460	188	272
Coffee or tea	0	0	0
Totals:	**460**	**188**	**272**

DINNER:

Subway's Red Wine Vinaigrette Club Sandwich (6")	350	139	211
Subway's vegetable beef soup (1 cup)	90	28	62
Subway's Veggie Delite salad	50	8	42
Subway's double chocolate cookie	209	45	164
Milk (1 cup)	150	0	150
Totals:	**849**	**220**	**629**
DAILY TOTALS:	**2,974**	**806**	**2,168**

SAMPLE WEIGHT LOSS MENU FOR A 62-YEAR-OLD, 194-POUND MALE GOURMAND (ALL MAIN COURSE DISHES ARE PROVIDED BY CHEF PHILIPPE BOULOT)

Goal Weight: 170 pounds

Target Weight Loss: 24 pounds, or 2 pounds per week, for 12 weeks

Basal Metabolic Rate: 2,142

Job Activity Level: Light Physically Active (score of 1.2)

After-Work Activity Level: Couch Potato (score of 0.00)

Exercise Activity Level: Moderately Active (Average 1 hour per day by playing 18 holes of golf without a cart, twice a week, averaging 3.5 hours per round)

Therefore, he needs 2,915 calories per day to maintain his body weight.

To lose 2 pounds per week, he must neutralize 7,000 starch calories per week, or about 1,000 starch calories per day.

After taking starch blockers, his total caloric intake is reduced to 1,915 calories per day.

FOOD	TOTAL CALORIES	NEUTRALIZED CALORIES	REMAINING CALORIES
BREAKFAST:			
Eggs Benedict (1 serving)	372	105	267
Shredded potatoes (2) cooked in 1 Tbsp oil	245	156	89
Fruit salad (1 cup), which includes strawberries, bananas, blueberries, peaches, and cantaloupe	155	32	123
Fresh orange juice (1 cup)	60	1	59
Totals:	**832**	**294**	**538**
SNACK:			
Fragrant Dilly Bread*	132	63	69

Cucumber slaw*	28	4	24
Mint herbal tea	0	0	0
Totals:	**160**	**67**	**93**

LUNCH:

Open-Faced Grilled Asparagus Sandwich* (an alternative could be a French Toasted Sandwich*, or broiled salmon)	270	64	206
Roasted Butternut Squash Soup*	112	8	104
Green salad with 1 Tbsp low-fat dressing	50	10	40
Whole Wheat Bread Sticks* (2)	120	76	44
Totals:	**552**	**158**	**394**

SNACK:

Sugar-syrup coated popcorn or "Kettle Corn" (1 cup)	135	49	86
Total:	**135**	**49**	**86**

DINNER:

Pinot Noir wine (1 glass)	74	0	74
Chicken Artichoke Hash with Poached Eggs and Tarragon Crème Fraîche* (an alternative could be a Dungeness Crab Club Sandwich*)	530	19	511
Vegetable Soup*	135	74	61
Potato Gnocchi*	298	163	135
Totals:	**1,079**	**256**	**823**
DAILY TOTALS:	**2,716**	**813**	**1,903**

SAMPLE WEIGHT LOSS MENU FOR A
48-YEAR-OLD, 250-POUND OBESE MALE

Goal Weight: 185 pounds

Target Weight Loss: 65 pounds, or 2 pounds per week, for 32 weeks

Basal Metabolic Rate: 2,820

Job Activity Level: Light Physically Active (score of 1.2)

After-Work Activity Level: Couch Potato (score of 0.00)

Exercise Activity Level: Light (15 minutes per day walking 2.5 m.p.h.)

Therefore, he needs 3,485 calories per day to maintain his body weight.

To lose 2 pounds per week, he must neutralize 7,000 starch calories per week, or about 1,000 starch calories per day.

After taking starch blockers, his total caloric intake is reduced to 2,485 calories per day.

FOOD	TOTAL CALORIES	NEUTRALIZED CALORIES	REMAINING CALORIES
BREAKFAST:			
2 poached eggs on 2 pieces toast (main course alternative: waffles, or cereal with milk)	290	105	185
Grapefruit with 1 tsp sugar	100	24	76
Fruit salad (1 cup), which includes strawberries, bananas, blueberries, peaches, and cantaloupe	155	32	123
Potato Pancake*	95	48	47
Coffee or herbal tea	0	0	0
Totals:	**640**	**209**	**431**
SNACK:			
Cheese crackers (10)	50	19	31
Iced tea with lemon (1 glass)	0	0	0
Totals:	**50**	**19**	**31**

LUNCH:

Macaroni and Cheese* (an alternative could be a Hot Turkey Sandwich*, or a tuna salad sandwich)	207	81	126
Beijing Pea Pod Salad*	168	0	42
Tomato soup (1 cup)	50	0	50
Saltine crackers (6)	105	79	26
Totals:	**530**	**160**	**244**

SNACK:

Cinnamon Crunch Bread* (1 slice)	211	92	119
Whole milk (1 cup)	150	0	150
Totals:	**361**	**92**	**269**

DINNER:

Imported beer (12 oz)	146	0	146
Chicken with Chanterelle Cream Sauce and Fettuccine* (an alternative could be Grilled Polenta with Piperade Basquaise*)	325	31	294
Mashed potatoes and gravy	340	188	152
Crunchy Apple Salad*	158	8	150
Homemade cream of mushroom soup	257	0	257
Totals:	**1,226**	**227**	**999**

DESSERT:

Rustic Butter Cake*	382	38	344
Cold chocolate milk (½ cup)	67	0	67
Totals:	**449**	**38**	**411**
DAILY TOTALS:	**3,256**	**745**	**2,385**

SAMPLE WEIGHT LOSS MENU FOR A 44-YEAR-OLD, 210-POUND OBESE FEMALE

Goal Weight: 145 pounds

Target Weight Loss: 65 pounds, or 2 pounds per week, for 33 weeks

Basal Metabolic Rate: 2,194

Job Activity Level: Sedentary (score of 1.1)

After-Work Activity Level: Go-getter (score of 0.02)

Exercise Activity Level: Moderate (30 minutes per day walking 2.5 m.p.h.)

Therefore, she needs 2,670 calories per day to maintain her body weight.

To lose 2 pounds per week, she must neutralize 7,000 starch calories per week, or about 1,000 starch calories per day.

After taking starch blockers, her total caloric intake is reduced to 1,670 calories per day.

FOOD	TOTAL CALORIES	NEUTRALIZED CALORIES	REMAINING CALORIES
BREAKFAST:			
Buckwheat pancakes (4), with 2 tsp butter and 3 Tbsp of maple syrup	368	140	228
Whole Wheat toast, 1 tsp butter	126	95	31
Sliced banana with 2 Tbsp honey-yogurt topping, 1 tsp crushed walnuts	143	20	123
Coffee or tea	0	0	0
Totals:	**637**	**255**	**382**
SNACK:			
Toasted bagel, both halves, with all-fruit jelly	210	80	130
Apple juice (1 cup)	106	2	104
Totals:	**316**	**82**	**234**

LUNCH:

Hot Turkey Sandwich* (an alternative could be Potato Soufflé*)	204	53	151
Potato chips (20)	220	80	140
Hearty Bean and Carrot Salad*	127	45	82
Totals:	**551**	**178**	**373**

SNACK:

Cornbread* (1 piece)	118	49	69
Chex™ mix (½ cup)	45	34	11
Apple (½)	45	9	36
Totals:	**208**	**92**	**116**

DINNER:

Broiled New York steak (4 oz) (an alternative could be Tahitian Chicken*, or poached Dover sole)	320	0	320
Dinner rolls (2) with 2 tsp whipped butter	246	180	66
Mashed potatoes with garlic butter (1 cup)	360	270	90
Corn on the cob (1)	100	63	37
Totals:	**1,026**	**513**	**513**
DAILY TOTALS:	**2,738**	**1,120**	**1,618**

SAMPLE WEIGHT MAINTENANCE MENU FOR A 41-YEAR-OLD, 128-POUND FEMALE WHO DESIRES MORE FOOD INTAKE

Goal Weight: maintain present weight

Target Weight Loss: none

Basal Metabolic Rate: 1,352

Job Activity Level: Light Physically Active (score of 1.2)

After-Work Activity Level: Go-getter (score of 0.02)

Exercise Activity Level: Active (45 minutes per day medium aerobics)

Therefore, she needs 1,867 calories per day to maintain her body weight.

FOOD	TOTAL CALORIES	NEUTRALIZED CALORIES	REMAINING CALORIES
BREAKFAST:			
All-Bran cereal (1 cup), with 1 sliced banana, 2 tsp brown sugar, and ½ cup skim milk	255	160	95
Whole wheat toast, 1 tsp butter (1 slice)	126	95	31
Totals:	**381**	**255**	**126**
SNACK:			
Toasted bagel (½) with a tomato slice and a slice of Cheddar cheese, with pepper	240	80	160
Fresh orange juice (1 cup)	60	1	59
Totals:	**300**	**81**	**219**
LUNCH:			
Bacon, lettuce, and tomato sandwich (an alternative could be an egg salad sandwich)	369	60	309

Oven-baked french fries (20)	340	160	180
Cold Potato Salad (Curry)*	205	92	113
Apple (1)	90	18	72
Totals:	**1,004**	**330**	**674**

SNACK:

Graham crackers (2)	60	23	37
Almonds (small portion)	32	0	32
Whole milk (1 cup)	150	0	150
Totals:	**242**	**23**	**219**

DINNER:

Italian Macaroni and Tomatoes* (an alternative could be smoked salmon with honey-mustard sauce)	230	100	130
Jalapeño Cornbread* (1 piece)	318	83	235
Manhattan Clam Chowder*	289	115	175
Red wine (1 glass)	74	0	74
Totals:	**911**	**298**	**614**
DAILY TOTALS:	**2,839**	**987**	**1,852**

TEN

RECIPES FOR THE STARCH BLOCKER DIET

Lose Fat—Not Flavor

To achieve complete success on the strategy, you must redistribute many of your daily calories to the starchy foods segment of the starch blocker diet. These starchy foods should be relatively low in fat and sugar, and high in protein, fiber, vitamins, and minerals. Many of the food items that fit this description are basic staples, and require minimal preparation and no recipes. This can include cereals, potatoes, rice, breads, lean meats, fish, and fresh fruits and vegetables.

However, most people get tired of a steady diet of staples, and often enjoy dining on more complex, varied dishes, which require a bit of preparation.

In this chapter, we provide you with a wealth of extremely tasty and nutritious dishes that will fit your starch blocker diet perfectly. They have been very carefully chosen to meet all the guidelines that determine appropriate strategy foods.

Many of these recipes are quite different from the types of recipes you generally see in weight loss books. They are generally more rich in starch than are most typical diet book recipes. If you were not taking starch blockers, you wouldn't be able to eat these high-starch dishes regularly. They'd be too fattening. Starch blockers, however, change everything. They allow you a freedom you've never before experienced on a diet.

By neutralizing starch calories, you not only enable yourself to freely eat starchy foods, but you also allow yourself to add some extra fat, sugar, and protein calories, to compensate in part for the starch calories you neutralize.

Therefore, you'll be able to feast on some very fanciful fare on this diet, such as Grilled Polenta with Piperade Basquaise, or Seafood Fettuccine Vin Blanc. Both of these recipes, and many others, come from famous French chef Philippe Boulot.

Chef of the award-winning Heathman Restaurant in Portland, Oregon, Philippe Boulot was the recipient of the 2001 James Beard Award for Best Chef in America, Northwest Region (including Hawaii). Formerly at Maxim's in Paris, The Mark Hotel Restaurant in New York, and The Clift in San Francisco, Chef Philippe was trained by the legendary French chefs Joel Robouchon and Alain Senderens, the originator of nouvelle cuisine. His recipes, as you'll note, are often rich and exotic. He cooks in the classic French style and strives to bring out flavors that will satisfy the soul as well as the palate. As you savor his creations—and still lose weight—you'll appreciate not only the artistry of this chef, but also the power of starch calorie neutralizaton. It opens a world of gourmet dining to people who, due to weight, may have long forgone its pleasures.

Many of the fine desserts and breads that we present were created by pastry chef Susan Boulot, Philippe's wife and a very prominent chef in her own right. A graduate of the Culinary Institute of America, in Hyde Park, New York, she was formerly the pastry chef at The Mark Hotel Restaurant and the Heathman Restaurant. Her culinary style is delicate, lush, and indulgent. Her desserts are a sensuous delight.

Many of the remaining recipes are hearty, tasty, traditional American home-cooking dishes. In essence, they are examples of the "American bistro" style—simple and satisfying family fare. If they remind you of Mom's home cooking, there's a reason: Many of the very best are taken directly from the files of Cameron Stauth's mother, Lorraine Stauth. Mrs. Stauth, formerly a broadcast journalist, had a cooking show of her own, but above all, her principal pride was in serving nourishing, satisfying, and delicious food to her own family.

Her recipes, carefully chosen for this book, realistically take into account the common family concerns of speed, ease, economy, and availability of ingredients. They also reflect the traditional American reliance upon wholesome, high-starch foods as a mainstay of the day-to-day diet.

Thus, you're provided here with a basic, nutritious meat-and-potatoes diet, adorned with a wide variety of the best of the world-class gourmet dishes that make dining fun and exciting.

These recipes will make your starch blocker diet a daily feast.

Most amazing of all, you *will* lose weight on this luscious, healthful new way of eating.

BREADS

CINNAMON CRUNCH BREAD
from the kitchen of chef Philippe Boulot

Ingredients	Calories	Blocked Starch Calories	Remaining Non-Starch Calories
1 cup milk	150	0	150
⅓ cup butter	542	0	542
2 packages dry active yeast	0	0	0
7 cups all-purpose flour	2800	2100	700
¾ cup plus 2 tablespoons sugar	630	0	630
1½ teaspoons salt	0	0	0
3 eggs, at room temperature	225	0	225
2 teaspoons cinnamon	0	0	0
1 egg white, slightly beaten	17	0	17
Crumb Topping:			
⅓ cup all-purpose flour	133	100	33
⅓ cup firmly packed brown sugar	267	0	267
1 teaspoon cinnamon	0	0	0
3 tablespoons butter	300	0	300

Combine the milk, ¾ cup water, and butter in a saucepan. Heat over low heat to body temperature or until lukewarm. The butter does not need to melt. Whisk in the yeast to dissolve. Let stand. Place 6 cups of the flour, sugar, and the salt in a mixing bowl. On low speed, gradually mix in the eggs, then the warm liquids, and incorporate all. Add the remaining flour slowly and mix, until the dough is no longer sticky. Knead for 10 minutes, or until the dough is smooth and elastic.

Place the dough in a lightly greased bowl, flipping the dough over to grease the top. Cover and let rise to double in size, 30 minutes to 1 hour.

Combine ½ cup sugar and the cinnamon in a small bowl and set aside. Punch down the dough and divide in half. Roll each half out to a 14 x 9-inch rectangle. Brush lightly with butter and sprinkle with the sugar and cinnamon mixture. Beginning at the short end, roll the dough tightly and shape into loaves, sealing the edges together. Place into a greased 9 x 5 x 3-inch pan, seam side down. Cover and allow to rise to double the size. Make the crumb topping: Combine the dry ingredients. Rub the butter into the topping mixture, until crumbly. Brush the loaves with egg white and sprinkle with the crumb topping.

    Bake in a 375°F oven, on the low rack, for about 15 minutes, or until the topping is set. Top the bread with a foil tent to prevent overbrowning. Bake another 45 minutes, and check to make sure it's done.

Makes 2 loaves, 12 slices each

TOTALS	PER RECIPE	PER LOAF	PER SLICE
Calories	5064	2532	211
Blocked Starch Calories	2200	1100	92
Remaining Non-Starch Calories	2864	1432	119

ANADAMA BREAD

INGREDIENTS	CALORIES	BLOCKED STARCH CALORIES	REMAINING NON-STARCH CALORIES
5½ to 6½ cups unsifted all-purpose flour	2400	1800	600
2½ teaspoons salt	0	0	0
1 cup yellow cornmeal	500	375	125
2 packages active dry yeast	0	0	0
¼ cup butter, softened	400	0	400
½ cup molasses, at room temperature	400	0	400

In a large bowl, thoroughly mix 2½ cups flour, the salt, cornmeal, yeast, and butter. Gradually add 2 cups hot water and the molasses. Beat with an electric mixer for 2 minutes at medium speed. Scraping the bowl occasionally, add ½ cup flour, or enough to make a stiff batter. Beat at high speed for 2 minutes. Stir in enough flour to make a soft dough. Place the dough on a floured board and knead for 8 to 10 minutes. Place in an oiled bowl and let rise until doubled in bulk, about 1 hour.

Punch the dough down and place on a floured board. Divide in half and shape into two loaves. Place in 2 oiled bread pans. Cover and let rise until doubled. Bake at 375°F for about 40 minutes or until done.

Makes 16 slices per loaf

TOTALS	PER RECIPE	PER LOAF	PER SLICE
Calories	3700	1850	116
Blocked Starch Calories	2175	1088	68
Remaining Non-Starch Calories	1525	763	48

JALAPEÑO CORNBREAD
from the kitchen of chef Philippe Boulot

INGREDIENTS	CALORIES	BLOCKED STARCH CALORIES	REMAINING NON-STARCH CALORIES
2 cups yellow or white cornmeal	960	720	240
2 cups all-purpose flour	800	600	200
½ cup sugar	360	0	360
½ teaspoon salt	0	0	0
1 tablespoon baking powder	0	0	0
2 cups buttermilk	198	0	198
2 eggs	150	0	150
1¼ cups butter, melted	2033	0	2033

¼ cup sour cream	123	0	123
1 cup grated cheddar cheese	450	0	450
1 jalapeño chile, minced	5	0	5
¼ cup finely chopped onion	15	2	13

Preheat the oven to 400°F. Combine the cornmeal, flour, sugar, salt, and baking powder in a mixing bowl. In another bowl, mix together the buttermilk, eggs, butter, and sour cream. Add to the dry ingredients and mix together. Add the cheese, chile, and onion and fold in, to blend.
Bake in a buttered 9 x 12-inch pan for 35 to 30 minutes.

Serves 16

TOTALS	PER RECIPE	PER SERVING
Calories	5094	318
Blocked Starch Calories	1322	83
Remaining Non-Starch Calories	3772	235

FRAGRANT DILLY BREAD
from the kitchen of chef Philippe Boulot

INGREDIENTS	CALORIES	BLOCKED STARCH CALORIES	REMAINING NON-STARCH CALORIES
2 packages active dry yeast	0	0	0
2 cups cottage cheese, slightly warmed	430	0	430
4 tablespoons sugar	180	0	180
½ teaspoon baking soda	0	0	0
1 tablespoon salt	0	0	0
1 teaspoon dried dill weed	0	0	0
1 teaspoon dill seed	0	0	0

2 eggs	150	0	150
4 tablespoons (½ stick) butter, softened, plus more for bowl and pan	407	0	407
5 cups all-purpose flour	2000	1500	500

Mix the yeast and ½ cup warm water (110° to 115°) in a large bowl, and let it sit until foamy, 3 to 5 minutes. Mix the slightly warm cottage cheese into the yeast and add the rest of the ingredients. Mix to make a soft dough, adjusting with more flour or water as needed. Knead until smooth and satiny. Let the dough rise in a greased bowl, covered with a damp cloth, until doubled in size.

Knead the dough lightly and divide it in half. Shape the dough into a tight ball and place it in a buttered 1½-quart casserole or a medium skillet, or leave it freeform on a greased baking pan. Cover with a damp cloth and let stand until doubled in size.

If desired, brush with a small quantity of a beaten egg and bake at 350°F for about 45 minutes.

Makes 2 loaves, 12 slices each

TOTALS	PER RECIPE	PER LOAF	PER SLICE
Calories	3167	1584	132
Blocked Starch Calories	1500	750	63
Remaining Non-Starch Calories	1667	834	69

BLUEBERRY CORNMEAL MUFFINS
from the kitchen of chef Philippe Boulot

INGREDIENTS	CALORIES	BLOCKED STARCH CALORIES	REMAINING NON-STARCH CALORIES
½ cup butter, softened	813	0	813
1 cup sugar	720	0	720

2 large eggs	150	0	150
1 teaspoon vanilla extract	0	0	0
2 teaspoons baking powder	0	0	0
¼ teaspoon salt	0	0	0
2½ cups blueberries	200	10	190
1½ cups all-purpose flour	600	450	150
½ cup yellow or white cornmeal	216	54	162
½ cup whole milk	75	0	75

Preheat the oven to 375°F. Cream the butter in a large bowl, adding the sugar slowly until light and fluffy. Beat in the eggs one at a time. Add the vanilla, baking powder, and salt. Mush ½ cup of the blueberries with a fork and add to batter. Fold in half of the flour, then half of the milk. Add the remaining flour and milk. Fold in the remaining blueberries. Scoop the batter into paper-lined muffin tins. Bake for 25 to 30 minutes, or until golden brown. Let the bread cool before removing from pans.

Serves 12

TOTALS	PER RECIPE	PER SERVING
Calories	2774	231
Blocked Starch Calories	514	43
Remaining Non-Starch Calories	2260	188

WHOLE WHEAT BREAD STICKS

INGREDIENTS	CALORIES	BLOCKED STARCH CALORIES	REMAINING NON-STARCH CALORIES
2 cups whole wheat flour	800	600	200
2 cups wheat germ	800	600	200

1¼ cups 2% milk	151	0	151
1 tablespoon safflower oil	115	0	115
1 tablespoon honey	61	0	61
1 teaspoon salt	0	0	0

Preheat the oven to 350°F. Mix the dry ingredients in a large bowl. Add the milk, oil, and honey. Mix well. Knead the dough in the bowl until it holds together well, about 10 minutes.

Place the dough on waxed paper on the counter or bread board and cut it into 32 pieces by first cutting into halves, then halving it again and again. Use your hands to roll the dough to about the size of a large pencil, 5 to 6 inches long. Place the bread sticks on nonstick baking sheets and bake for 30 to 40 minutes, or until firm and lightly browned.

Makes 32 bread sticks

TOTALS	PER RECIPE	PER STICK
Calories	1927	60
Blocked Starch Calories	1200	38
Remaining Non-Starch Calories	727	23

CORNBREAD

INGREDIENTS	CALORIES	BLOCKED STARCH CALORIES	REMAINING NON-STARCH CALORIES
4 tablespoons butter, melted	280	0	280
1⅓ tablespoons honey	81	0	81
2 eggs, beaten	150	0	150
1 cup 2% milk	121	0	121
1 cup yellow or white cornmeal	380	285	95

1 cup all-purpose flour	400	300	100
2 teaspoons baking powder	0	0	0
1 teaspoon salt	0	0	0

Combine all the ingredients in a large bowl, beating only slightly. Pour the batter into a well-oiled pan and bake at 375°F for 25 to 30 minutes.

Makes 12 squares

TOTALS	PER RECIPE	PER SERVING
Calories	1412	118
Blocked Starch Calories	585	49
Remaining Non-Starch Calories	827	69

BANANA NUT BREAD

INGREDIENTS	CALORIES	BLOCKED STARCH CALORIES	REMAINING NON-STARCH CALORIES
2 eggs	160	0	160
⅔ cup honey	650	0	650
⅓ cup safflower oil	640	0	640
1 cup mashed bananas	240	180	60
1 teaspoon baking soda	0	0	0
½ teaspoon baking powder	0	0	0
2¼ cups all-purpose flour	900	675	225
Pinch of salt	0	0	0
½ cup chopped nuts	400	0	400

Preheat oven to 350°F. Beat the eggs in a large bowl; add honey and mix. Combine the oil, bananas, baking soda, and baking powder. Add the bananas to the eggs, alternating with the flour and salt. Add the nuts. Bake for 45 to 50 minutes.

Serves 20

TOTALS	PER RECIPE	PER SERVING
Calories	2990	150
Blocked Starch Calories	855	43
Remaining Non-Starch Calories	2135	107

HEAVENLY BISCUITS

INGREDIENTS	CALORIES	BLOCKED STARCH CALORIES	REMAINING NON-STARCH CALORIES
1 package dry yeast	0	0	0
2½ cups all-purpose flour	1000	750	250
½ teaspoon baking soda	0	0	0
1 teaspoon baking powder	0	0	0
1 teaspoon salt	0	0	0
1 tablespoon honey	40	0	40
2 tablespoons butter	200	0	200
1 cup buttermilk	90	0	90
Vegetable oil spray for pan	0	0	0

Dissolve the yeast in ¼ cup warm water (110° to 115°), with honey. Mix the dry ingredients and cut in butter, as you would for pie dough. Add buttermilk and yeast mixture. Knead lightly on floured board. Roll out and cut into 1"–2" high biscuits with a biscuit cutter or a glass. Place on an oiled pan, cover, and let rise for about 1 hour. Preheat oven to 350°F, and bake about 20 minutes, or until nicely browned.

Makes 12

TOTALS	PER RECIPE	PER SERVING
Calories	1330	111
Blocked Starch Calories	750	63
Remaining Non-Starch Calories	580	48

POPOVERS

INGREDIENTS	CALORIES	BLOCKED STARCH CALORIES	REMAINING NON-STARCH CALORIES
2 eggs, beaten	150	0	150
1 cup whole milk	150	0	150
1 tablespoon oil	125	0	125
1 cup all-purpose flour, sifted	400	300	100
¼ teaspoon salt	0	0	0
Vegetable oil spray for baking cups	0	0	0

Preheat the oven to 450°F. Place all the ingredients in a blender, and mix until well blended. Oil heavy baking cups, and heat them in the oven before filling them half full with popover batter. Bake about 30 minutes. Turn the oven down to 350°F, and bake another 15 minutes. Great for breakfast or with fruit salad for lunch.

Makes 8 to 10

TOTALS	PER RECIPE	PER SERVING (8)	PER SERVING (10)
Calories	825	103	83
Blocked Starch Calories	300	38	30
Remaining Non-Starch Calories	525	65	53

POTATOES

LYONNAISE POTATOES
from the kitchen of chef Philippe Boulot

Ingredients	Calories	Blocked Starch Calories	Remaining Non-Starch Calories
¼ cup chopped onions	15	2	13
1 clove garlic	0	0	0
1 tablespoon olive oil	125	0	125
1 pound small fingerling potatoes	440	70	370
1 cup chicken stock	15	0	15
1 sprig thyme	0	0	0
1 sprig rosemary	0	0	0
Salt and freshly ground pepper	0	0	0

Sauté the onions and garlic slowly in the olive oil, until caramelized. Add the potatoes, stock, herbs, and some salt and pepper. Cover and simmer slowly until the potatoes are tender, about ½ hour.

Serves 4

Totals	Per Recipe	Per Serving
Calories	595	149
Blocked Starch Calories	72	18
Remaining Non-Starch Calories	523	131

POTATO GNOCCHI
from the kitchen of chef Philippe Boulot

Ingredients	Calories	Blocked Starch Calories	Remaining Non-Starch Calories
2 large russet or baking potatoes	240	52	188
Salt			
2 cups all-purpose flour, plus more for dusting	800	600	200
2 eggs	150	0	150
1 teaspoon freshly ground pepper	0	0	0
1 teaspoon freshly ground nutmeg	0	0	0

Preheat the oven to 375°F. Peel and cut the potatoes into large chunks. Place them in a saucepan and cover with water; add salt, and cook until potatoes are tender. Drain and spread out on a baking pan. Let dry in the oven for 10 minutes. Pass the potatoes through a food mill or ricer, directly onto a lightly floured table or cutting board. Make a well in the center, and add the eggs, salt, pepper, and nutmeg. Sprinkle with the flour and slowly work together to make a smooth, slightly sticky dough. Don't overknead the dough, as this will make it tough.

Divide the dough into 4 pieces and roll each into a ¾-inch-diameter rope, using only enough extra flour to keep it from sticking. Cut the rope into ½-inch pieces. The gnocchi can be cooked as is, or shaped by rolling the pieces over the floured tines of a fork. Bring a large pot of water to a boil with some salt. Drop the gnocchi in and simmer until they rise to the surface, about 5 minutes. Skim them off and drain in a colander. You can sauté the gnocchi or toss in melted butter, adding Parmesan cheese and some herbs. The gnocchi can also be tossed into a light tomato sauce.

Serves 4

Totals	Per Recipe	Per Serving
Calories	1190	298
Blocked Starch Calories	652	163
Remaining Non-Starch Calories	538	135

POTATO KUGEL

Ingredients	Calories	Blocked Starch Calories	Remaining Non-Starch Calories
8 large potatoes	1160	870	290
1 large onion	35	3	32
4 carrots	140	12	128
2 eggs, beaten	150	0	150
½ cup whole wheat breadcrumbs	150	113	37
1 tablespoon all-purpose flour	25	19	6
1 teaspoon celery salt	0	0	0
Freshly ground pepper	0	0	0

Preheat oven to 375°F. Grate the potatoes, onion, and carrots into a bowl. Drain off any liquid. Mix the eggs with the breadcrumbs, flour, celery salt, and pepper and add to the vegetable mixture. Place in an oiled casserole dish or 8 x 8-inch pan and bake for 1 hour, or until the top is crusted and the vegetables are tender.

Serves 4 to 6

Totals	Per Recipe	Per serving (4)	Per serving (6)
Calories	1660	415	277
Blocked Starch Calories	1017	254	170
Remaining Non-Starch Calories	643	161	107

SCALLOPED POTATOES AU GRATIN

Ingredients	Calories	Blocked Starch Calories	Remaining Non-Starch Calories
3 tablespoons whipped butter, plus more for dish	210	0	210
2 tablespoons all-purpose flour	50	38	12
2 cups hot whole milk	300	0	300
Salt and freshly ground pepper	0	0	0
½ cup Cheddar cheese	225	0	225
6 medium potatoes, sliced	720	540	180
1 onion, chopped (optional)	35	3	32

Preheat the oven to 375°F. Melt the butter in a heavy-bottomed skillet on low heat. Stir in the flour until smooth. Add the milk gradually, stirring continually, until well blended. Add the cheese to the mixture. Layer the sliced potatoes, onions, and cheese sauce in a buttered baking dish. Season with salt and pepper. Cover, and bake for about 45 minutes. Remove cover and bake 15 minutes more.

Serves 6

Totals	Per Recipe	Per Serving
Calories	1540	257
Blocked Starch Calories	581	97
Remaining Non-Starch Calories	959	160

POTATO PANCAKES

Ingredients	Calories	Blocked Starch Calories	Remaining Non-Starch Calories
6 medium potatoes, peeled	720	540	180
1 onion	35	3	32
4 slices bacon	180	0	180
2 tablespoons all-purpose flour	50	38	12
1 tablespoon chopped flat-leaf parsley	0	0	0
2 eggs, beaten	160	0	160
Salt and freshly ground pepper	0	0	0

Grate the potatoes and onion, and drain off the juice. Fry the bacon in a nonstick skillet until crisp. Remove the bacon and crumble, leaving the fat in the skillet to fry the potato pancakes. Mix the grated potatoes and onion with the flour and bacon bits. Add the chopped parsley, eggs, salt, and pepper. Heat the bacon fat, and pour about ⅓ cup of batter into it for each pancake. When the pancakes are brown on bottom, turn them over and brown the other side. When they're done, place them on paper towels to drain. If preferred, olive oil may be used instead of bacon fat.

Makes about 12

Totals	Per Recipe	Per Serving
Calories	1145	95
Blocked Starch Calories	581	48
Remaining Non-Starch Calories	564	47

YAM FLUFF

Ingredients	Calories	Blocked Starch Calories	Remaining Non-Starch Calories
4 medium-sized yams	720	540	180
½ cup orange juice	60	0	60
1½ tablespoons honey	97	0	97
½ teaspoon salt	0	0	0
¼ cup sunflower seeds	187	0	187
Vegetable oil spray, for dish	0	0	0

Preheat oven to 375°F. Bake yams in oven, or microwave, until they're soft. Peel the yams and put them in a bowl. Add orange juice, honey, and salt, and whip with an electric hand-mixer until fluffy. Mix in half of the sunflower seeds. Spoon yams into a buttered casserole dish, and top with remainder of seeds. Bake for about 30 minutes.

Serves 6

Totals	Per Recipe	Per Serving
Calories	1064	177
Blocked Starch Calories	540	90
Remaining Non-Starch Calories	524	87

COLD POTATO SALAD (CURRY)

Ingredients	Calories	Blocked Starch Calories	Remaining Non-Starch Calories
4 medium-size potatoes, cooked in skins or baked, then peeled and diced	480	360	120
½ cup diced celery	10	3	7
¼ cup diced cucumber	15	0	15
1 tablespoon finely chopped green pepper	5	2	3
2 hard-boiled eggs, chopped	150	0	150
4 scallions or 1 onion, diced	35	3	32
1 tablespoon vinegar	0	0	0
1 tablespoon sugar	45	0	45
½ cup prepared low-calorie mayonnaise	80	0	80
1 tablespoon curry powder (optional)	0	0	0
Salt and freshly ground pepper	0	0	0
Lettuce	0	0	0
Paprika	0	0	0

Place all the ingredients in a bowl, and mix thoroughly. Chill before serving. Serve the salad on a lettuce leaf and sprinkle with dash of paprika.

Serves 4

Totals	Per Recipe	Per Serving
Calories	820	205
Blocked Starch Calories	368	92
Remaining Non-Starch Calories	452	113

POTATO SOUFFLÉ

Ingredients	Calories	Blocked Starch Calories	Remaining Non-Starch Calories
6 medium potatoes, peeled	960	720	240
½ cup whole milk	75	0	75
1 tablespoon whipped butter, plus more for dish	70	0	70
2 eggs, separated	150	0	150
Salt and freshly ground pepper	0	0	0

Preheat oven to 375°F. Cook the potatoes in boiling water until tender. Drain. Add the milk, butter, egg yolks, salt, and pepper, and mash until light and fluffy. Beat the egg whites with an electric hand-mixer until stiff, and fold into the potato mixture. Place the potatoes in a buttered baking dish and bake for about 30 minutes. Serve immediately.

Serves 4

Totals	Per Recipe	Per Serving
Calories	1255	314
Blocked Starch Calories	720	180
Remaining Non-Starch Calories	535	134

SOUPS

MANHATTAN CLAM CHOWDER

Ingredients	Calories	Blocked Starch Calories	Remaining Non-Starch Calories
2 slices bacon, diced	90	0	90
2 tablespoons minced onion	15	1	14
2 seven-ounce cans minced or whole clams	252	0	252
2 cups cooked tomatoes	120	0	120
½ cup diced celery	10	3	7
2 cups diced potatoes	600	450	150
1 cup diced carrots	70	6	64
Salt	0	0	0
Pinch of rosemary	0	0	0
Pinch of thyme	0	0	0

Fry the bacon and brown the onion in the fat. Add the liquid from the clams, plus about ½ cup of water and the 2 cups cooked tomatoes. Bring to a boil and add the celery, potatoes, carrots, salt, rosemary, and thyme. Cook until the vegetables are tender. Just before serving, add the tomatoes and clams. Reheat and serve.

Serves 4

Totals	Per Recipe	Per Serving
Calories	1157	289
Blocked Starch Calories	460	115
Remaining Non-Starch Calories	697	175

ROASTED BUTTERNUT SQUASH SOUP
from the kitchen of chef Philippe Boulot

Ingredients	Calories	Blocked Starch Calories	Remaining Non-Starch Calories
1 pound 4 ounces butternut squash	45	8	37
2 slices bacon, diced	78	0	78
1 cup diced carrot	70	6	64
1 cup diced onion	54	4	50
1 cup diced celery	20	6	14
2 garlic cloves, chopped	0	0	0
4 cups chicken stock	60	0	60
1 cup apple cider	116	8	108
1 tablespoon lemon juice	4	1	3
¼ teaspoon cinnamon	0	0	0
Pinch of nutmeg	0	0	0
Pinch of cloves	0	0	0
Salt and freshly ground pepper	0	0	0
Bouquet garni: small sprigs of parsley and thyme tied together with a piece of bay leaf	0	0	0

Preheat oven to 400°F. Peel and seed the squash. Cut into chunks. Spread out on a baking sheet and roast for 15 to 20 minutes. Shake the pan and turn the pieces over, and continue baking until squash is completely tender, 30 to 45 minutes.

Cook the bacon in a large stockpot. Add the carrot, onion, celery, and garlic to the pot, cooking until soft. Add the prepared squash, the stock, and cider. Bring to a simmer and add lemon juice, cinnamon, nutmeg, cloves, salt, pepper, and bouquet garni. Cook for 30 minutes until the flavors are well blended. Remove the bouquet garni and puree the soup smooth with an immersion blender.

Serves 4

Totals	Per Recipe	Per Serving
Calories	447	112
Blocked Starch Calories	33	8
Remaining Non-Starch Calories	414	104

GOOD OLD-FASHIONED POTATO SOUP

Ingredients	Calories	Blocked Starch Calories	Remaining Non-Starch Calories
4 cooked, mashed potatoes, cooking water reserved	480	360	120
1 cup whole milk	150	0	150
1 tablespoon whipped butter	70	0	70
Salt and freshly ground pepper	0	0	0
2 teaspoons diced onion	0	0	0
Paprika	0	0	0

Combine 1 cup potato liquid and the milk in a stockpot. Add the mashed potatoes; heat until simmering. Add the butter, salt, and pepper. Add ½ teaspoon diced, raw onion to each bowl, pour in the soup, and sprinkle with paprika.

Serves 4

Totals	Per Recipe	Per Serving
Calories	700	175
Blocked Starch Calories	360	90
Remaining Non-Starch Calories	340	85

QUICK CHICKEN NOODLE SOUP

Ingredients	Calories	Blocked Starch Calories	Remaining Non-Starch Calories
4 cups chicken broth	120	0	120
½ cup diced celery	10	3	7
½ cup diced carrots	35	3	32
1 tablespoon minced onion	8	0	8
2 cups cooked whole wheat, spinach, or plain noodles	400	300	100
Minced parsley	0	0	0

Bring the chicken broth to a boil. Add the vegetables and noodles, and cook until tender, about 15 minutes. Season as desired. Pour the soup in bowls and sprinkle with minced parsley.

Serves 4

Totals	Per Recipe	Per Serving
Calories	573	143
Blocked Starch Calories	306	77
Remaining Non-Starch Calories	267	66

SPLIT PEA OR NAVY BEAN SOUP

Ingredients	Calories	Blocked Starch Calories	Remaining Non-Starch Calories
2 cups dried split peas or navy beans	1050	788	262
1 minced onion	35	3	32
2 stalks celery, minced	20	6	14

	Calories	Blocked Starch Calories	Remaining Non-Starch Calories
1 carrot, diced fine	35	3	32
½ pound finely diced ham (optional)	480	0	480
Salt and freshly ground pepper	0	0	0
Minced parsley	0	0	0

Soak the peas or navy beans in 3 quarts water overnight. Add the vegetables and cook slowly for about 3 hours, or until the beans are tender and the liquid is cooked down to consistency you like. Add the diced ham, if using. Season with salt, pepper, and minced parsley. If you prefer a smooth pea soup, run it through a blender before you add the ham cubes.

Serves 8

TOTALS	PER RECIPE	PER SERVING
Calories	1620	203
Blocked Starch Calories	800	100
Remaining Non-Starch Calories	820	103

WESTERN CHILI

INGREDIENTS	CALORIES	BLOCKED STARCH CALORIES	REMAINING NON-STARCH CALORIES
½ pound ground round (or extra-lean hamburger)	425	0	425
1 onion, chopped	35	3	32
2 green bell peppers, chopped coarsely	32	0	32
2 sixteen-ounce cans hot chili beans	1120	840	280
1 teaspoon sugar	15	0	15
2 sixteen-ounce cans tomatoes	120	0	120
1 teaspoon hot green salsa	0	0	0
Salt and freshly ground pepper	0	0	0

Mix the beef, onion, and bell pepper in a nonstick skillet and stir until browned. Mix the meat mixture with the remaining ingredients and simmer, covered, for about 1 hour, or cook in slow cooker or crock pot according to directions.

Makes 6 large bowls or 8 medium ones

TOTALS	PER RECIPE	PER SERVING (6)	PER SERVING (8)
Calories	1747	291	218
Blocked Starch Calories	843	141	105
Remaining Non-Starch Calories	904	150	113

VEGETABLE SOUP

INGREDIENTS	CALORIES	BLOCKED STARCH CALORIES	REMAINING NON-STARCH CALORIES
2 cups diced potatoes	540	405	135
1 cup sliced carrots	70	6	64
1 cup sliced celery	10	6	4
1 onion, chopped	35	3	32
4 cups tomatoes	240	0	240
2 cups shredded cabbage	34	0	34
1 cup uncooked macaroni	420	315	105
1 tablespoon chopped parsley	0	0	0
Salt and freshly ground pepper	0	0	0

Place the potatoes, carrots, celery, onion, and 2 cups water in large saucepan and cook about 15 minutes. Add remaining ingredients and simmer, covered, until the macaroni is tender.

Serves 8 to 10

TOTALS	PER RECIPE	PER SERVING (8)	PER SERVING (10)
Calories	1349	169	135
Blocked Starch Calories	735	92	74
Remaining Non-Starch Calories	614	77	61

HEARTY BARLEY SOUP

INGREDIENTS	CALORIES	BLOCKED STARCH CALORIES	REMAINING NON-STARCH CALORIES
1½ cups barley	1140	855	285
1 onion, chopped	35	3	32
2 carrots, chopped	70	6	64
1 stalk sliced celery	10	3	7
2 beef bouillon cubes	10	0	10
1 cup tomatoes	60	0	60
Salt and freshly ground pepper	0	0	0

Combine all the ingredients plus 4 cups water in a large saucepan. Bring to a boil, turn down heat, cover, and simmer for about 1 hour, or until the soup reaches desired consistency. Season with sea or celery salt and pepper.

Serves 4

TOTALS	PER RECIPE	PER SERVING
Calories	1325	331
Blocked Starch Calories	867	217
Remaining Non-Starch Calories	458	114

SANDWICHES

OPEN-FACED GRILLED ASPARAGUS SANDWICH
from the kitchen of chef Philippe Boulot

Ingredients	Calories	Blocked Starch Calories	Remaining Non-Starch Calories
1 pound fresh asparagus, trimmed and washed	60	16	44
Extra-virgin olive oil, plus more for bread	30	0	0
4 pieces artisan olive bread	380	240	140
Relish (optional)			
8 ounces sliced smoked mozzarella	640	0	640
Salt and freshly ground pepper	0	0	0

Heat a grill or grill pan until hot. Toss the asparagus in olive oil. Grill the asparagus spears. Lightly brush the bread with about ¼ teaspoon of olive oil and quickly grill until toasted, but not dry, on both sides. Spread with some relish, if desired. Lay the asparagus spears generously on the bread and arrange the slices of cheese over them. Put the sandwiches under the broiler until the cheese melts.

Serves 4

Totals	Per Recipe	Per Serving
Calories	1110	277
Blocked Starch Calories	256	64
Remaining Non-Starch Calories	854	213

HOT CRAB SANDWICH

Ingredients	Calories	Blocked Starch Calories	Remaining Non-Starch Calories
2 English muffins	280	210	70
1 cup crabmeat	156	0	156
¼ cup diced celery	5	2	3
2 tablespoons diced green pepper	5	0	5
1 tablespoon diced onion	8	0	8
1 teaspoon lemon juice	0	0	0
4 tablespoons low-calorie mayonnaise	100	0	100

Preheat the broiler. Split English muffins, toast them, and set aside. Shred the crabmeat, and mix with the celery, green pepper, onion, lemon juice, and mayonnaise. Spread the crab mixture on the muffins and place under the broiler until heated through.

Serves 4

Totals	Per Recipe	Per Serving
Calories	554	139
Blocked Starch Calories	212	53
Remaining Non-Starch Calories	342	86

EGG SALAD SANDWICH

Ingredients	Calories	Blocked Starch Calories	Remaining Non-Starch Calories
6 eggs, hard-boiled	550	0	550
1 tablespoon minced onion	8	0	8

¼ cup minced celery	5	2	3
1 tablespoon pickle relish	4	1	3
½ teaspoon dry mustard	0	0	0
½ teaspoon curry powder	0	0	0
½ cup low-calorie sandwich spread	40	30	10
8 slices whole wheat or rye bread	880	660	220
Salt	0	0	0

Peel and chop the eggs, and combine them with the remaining ingredients except the bread; mix well, adding salt to taste. Chill the salad. Divide the salad among 4 slices of bread, and cover with remaining slices.

Serves 4

TOTALS	PER RECIPE	PER SERVING
Calories	1487	372
Blocked Starch Calories	693	173
Remaining Non-Starch Calories	794	199

CROQUE MONSIEUR
from the kitchen of chef Philippe Boulot

INGREDIENTS	CALORIES	BLOCKED STARCH CALORIES	REMAINING NON-STARCH CALORIES
1 ounce butter	203	0	203
¼ cup all-purpose flour	100	75	25
2 cups whole milk	300	0	300
1 cup grated Gruyère or Emmenthal cheese	760	0	760
1 cup grated Parmesan cheese	455	0	455
1 fresh crusty baguette	600	450	150

12 ounces ham, sliced	828	0	828
8 ounces Swiss cheese, sliced	856	0	856
Salt and freshly ground pepper	0	0	0

Preheat the oven to 350°F. Melt the butter in a small saucepan. When it starts to bubble, add the flour, and stir. On low heat, let it cook gently for a few minutes. It should not brown. Slowly whisk in the milk, avoiding lumps. Let this cook very gently for 5 minutes. Stir in the Gruyère and Parmesan cheeses, and adjust the seasoning. Place to the side, off the heat. Split the baguette up into 6 pieces and cut them in half, horizontally. Spread both sides generously with some sauce and layer on first the ham slices, then the Swiss cheese. Put on a baking sheet and place in oven until heated through and bubbling.

Serves 6

TOTALS	PER RECIPE	PER SERVING
Calories	4342	724
Blocked Starch Calories	525	88
Remaining Non-Starch Calories	3817	636

HOT TURKEY SANDWICH

INGREDIENTS	CALORIES	BLOCKED STARCH CALORIES	REMAINING NON-STARCH CALORIES
2 English muffins	280	210	70
4 slices turkey, 2 ounces each	400	0	400
1 medium dill pickle	5	1	4
½ cup mushroom soup	130	0	130

Split the English muffins. Toast them and set aside. Slice the dill pickle. Place a slice of turkey on each muffin, and top with pickle slices and 2 tablespoons mushroom soup. Place under the broiler until hot.

Serves 4

TOTALS	PER RECIPE	PER SERVING
Calories	815	204
Blocked Starch Calories	211	53
Remaining Non-Starch Calories	604	151

FRENCH TOASTED SANDWICH

INGREDIENTS	CALORIES	BLOCKED STARCH CALORIES	REMAINING NON-STARCH CALORIES
4 tablespoons low-calorie mayonnaise	100	0	100
1 teaspoon salad mustard	80	0	80
8 slices whole wheat bread	880	660	220
4 slices chicken or turkey	320	0	320
½ cup 2% milk	60	0	60
Vegetable oil spray	0	0	0

Mix the mayonnaise and mustard together and spread on the bread. Divide the slices of chicken or turkey among 4 pieces of bread and top with remaining slices. Mix the egg and milk together, and dip each side of the sandwich into the mixture just long enough to coat (do not soak). Spray the saucepan with vegetable oil and brown the sandwiches over low heat.

Serves 4

TOTALS	PER RECIPE	PER SERVING
Calories	1440	360
Blocked Starch Calories	660	165
Remaining Non-Starch Calories	780	195

ENGLISH VEGETARIAN SANDWICH

Ingredients	Calories	Blocked Starch Calories	Remaining Non-Starch Calories
2 English muffins	280	210	70
½ green pepper, diced	8	0	8
1 small onion, sliced	27	2	25
8 mushrooms, sliced	30	0	30
1 large tomato, sliced thin	35	0	35
2 tablespoons our low-calorie sandwich spread (see page 255)	10	0	10
Sea salt and freshly ground pepper	0	0	0
4 slices Cheddar cheese	400	0	400

Preheat the broiler. Split the English muffins, toast them, and set aside. In a small amount of boiling, salted water, parboil the pepper, onion, and mushrooms for about 5 minutes; drain. Spread each of the toasted muffins with sandwich spread, and cover them with slices of tomato, then onions, mushrooms, and green pepper, and a slice of cheese. Place under the broiler until the cheese is melted and bubbly.

Serves 4

Totals	Per Recipe	Per Serving
Calories	790	198
Blocked Starch Calories	212	53
Remaining Non-Starch Calories	578	145

DUNGENESS CRAB CLUB SANDWICH
from the kitchen of chef Philippe Boulot

Ingredients	Calories	Blocked Starch Calories	Remaining Non-Starch Calories
¼ cup pasteurized egg yolks	118	0	118
2 tablespoons fresh lemon juice	8	2	6
1 tablespoon chili-garlic paste	0	0	0
1 tablespoon Dijon mustard	10	0	10
Salt and freshly ground pepper	0	0	0
¾ cup extra-virgin olive oil	1432	0	1432
10 ounces fresh Dungeness crabmeat	255	0	255
¼ cup diced fennel	7	0	7
¼ cup chopped red onion	15	2	13
¼ cup chopped celery	5	2	3
8 slices smoked bacon, cooked	312	0	312
2 ripe tomatoes, sliced	52	0	52
12 slices lightly toasted brioche	640	480	160

Combine the egg yolks, lemon juice, chili paste, mustard, salt, and pepper in a mixing bowl. Whisk to combine, and add olive oil slowly, whisking vigorously to make a thick aioli (a thick and aromatic mayonnaise). This can also be done in a food processor or blender. Place the crabmeat, fennel, onion, and celery in a bowl. Fold enough aioli into the crabmeat mixture to make a creamy, flavorful filling. Divide the crab filling among 4 slices of brioche, and place another slice on top. Lay the bacon and tomato slices on the second layer, and top with remaining slices of brioche.

Serves 4

Totals	Per Recipe	Per Serving
Calories	2854	714
Blocked Starch Calories	486	122
Remaining Non-Starch Calories	2368	592

LOW-CALORIE STARCHY MAYONNAISE SUBSTITUTE

Ingredients	Calories	Blocked Starch Calories	Remaining Non-Starch Calories
1 fourteen-and-a-half-ounce can chicken broth	30	0	30
3 tablespoons cornstarch	90	68	22
1 tablespoon lemon juice	4	1	3
1 tablespoon grated onion	8	0	8
1 clove garlic, minced (optional)	0	0	0

Place about 6 tablespoons of the chicken broth and the cornstarch in a bowl and mix to combine. Combine the remaining broth, the lemon juice, grated onion, and garlic in a saucepan and bring to a boil. Add the cornstarch mixture to thicken. If no other seasonings are to be added, cool the mayonnaise, place it in covered jar, and refrigerate at least 1 hour.

Makes approximately 1½ cups

Totals	Per Recipe	Per serving (1 tablespoon)
Calories	132	7
Blocked Starch Calories	69	3
Remaining Non-Starch Calories	63	4

SALADS AND SALAD DRESSINGS

CRUNCHY APPLE SALAD

Ingredients	Calories	Blocked Starch Calories	Remaining Non-Starch Calories
4 medium apples, diced	360	24	336
1 cup red grapes	120	0	120
1 cup diced celery	20	6	14
½ cup of sweetened yogurt	130	0	130
Cherries or mint sprigs	0	0	0

Core, peel, and dice the apples. Halve the grapes and remove seeds. Mix all the ingredients together, and serve on lettuce tops. Garnish with cherry or sprig of mint.

Serves 4

Totals	Per Recipe	Per serving (1 tablespoon)
Calories	630	158
Blocked Starch Calories	30	8
Remaining Non-Starch Calories	600	150

HEARTY BEAN AND CARROT SALAD

Ingredients	Calories	Blocked Starch Calories	Remaining Non-Starch Calories
1 cup green beans, steamed	30	0	30
1 cup sliced carrots	70	6	64
1 cup canned red kidney beans	220	165	55
1 onion, sliced	35	3	32
½ cup chopped celery	10	3	7
1 green pepper, chopped	16	0	16
1 tablespoon sunflower seeds	45	0	45
½ cup low-calorie Italian salad dressing	80	0	80
Cherry tomatoes	0	0	0

Mix all the ingredients together and let stand at room temperature for about 1 hour before serving. Divide among 4 lettuce cups and garnish with a cherry tomato.

Serves 4

Totals	Per Recipe	Per Serving
Calories	506	127
Blocked Starch Calories	177	45
Remaining Non-Starch Calories	329	82

BEIJING PEA POD SALAD

Ingredients	Calories	Blocked Starch Calories	Remaining Non-Starch Calories
1 cup snow peas	70	0	70
Salt	0	0	0
1 cup shredded Chinese cabbage	30	0	30
¼ cup bamboo shoots	20	0	20
4 water chestnuts, sliced	20	0	20
4 mushrooms, sliced	20	0	20
1 tablespoon lemon juice	4	0	4
2 teaspoons soy sauce	4	0	4
½ teaspoon dry mustard	0	0	0
Cherry tomatoes	0	0	0

Cook the snow peas in boiling, salted water until tender and chill in the refrigerator. Combine the pea pods with the other vegetables. Mix the lemon juice, soy sauce, and mustard. Pour the dressing over the vegetables and toss well. Garnish with cherry tomatoes.

Serves 4

Totals	Per Recipe	Per Serving
Calories	168	42
Blocked Starch Calories	0	0
Remaining Non-Starch Calories	168	42

CUCUMBER SLAW

Ingredients	Calories	Blocked Starch Calories	Remaining Non-Starch Calories
3 cups grated green cabbage	51	24	27
1 cucumber, grated	30	0	30
1 green pepper, grated	16	0	16
1 tablespoon grated onion	8	0	8
½ cup creamy dill salad dressing	65	0	65
Cherry tomatoes, or paprika	0	0	0

Combine the vegetables and toss with a dill dressing. Serve on lettuce leaves and garnish with cherry tomatoes, or sprinkle with paprika.

Serves 6

Totals	Per Recipe	Per Serving
Calories	170	28
Blocked Starch Calories	24	4
Remaining Non-Starch Calories	146	24

RED KIDNEY BEAN SALAD

Ingredients	Calories	Blocked Starch Calories	Remaining Non-Starch Calories
1 can kidney beans (2 cups), drained	1056	792	264
¼ cup white vinegar	4	0	4
3 tablespoons safflower oil	360	0	360
½ cup diced celery	10	3	7
3 tablespoons chopped onion	23	2	21
2 tablespoons sugar	90	0	90
1 egg, hard-boiled and diced	80	0	80
½ teaspoon dry mustard	0	0	0

Combine all the ingredients and chill. Serve the salad on lettuce cups.

Serves 4

Totals	Per Recipe	Per Serving
Calories	1623	405
Blocked Starch Calories	797	199
Remaining Non-Starch Calories	826	206

STARCHY SALAD DRESSING

Ingredients	Calories	Blocked Starch Calories	Remaining Non-Starch Calories
½ cup juice from kosher dill pickles	0	0	0
1 tablespoon cornstarch	30	23	7
1 tablespoon finely diced onion	8	0	8
1 tablespoon finely diced cucumber	5	0	5
1 tablespoon finely diced carrot	3	0	3
Celery salt	0	0	0

Combine the pickle juice with ½ cup water. Mix 2 tablespoons of the pickle juice with the cornstarch to make a paste. Heat the remainder of the juice and thicken with the cornstarch paste, stirring it in slowly after the juice comes to a boil. If any lumps form, strain them out. Allow to cool, then add the vegetables. Season to taste with celery salt. Store the dressing in a covered container in the refrigerator. Stir before serving. If the dressing is too thick, add a little pickle juice. This is great on any kind of vegetable salad.

Serves 6

Totals	Per Recipe	Per Serving
Calories	46	7
Blocked Starch Calories	23	4
Remaining Non-Starch Calories	23	3

RICE

GINGER RICE

Ingredients	Calories	Blocked Starch Calories	Remaining Non-Starch Calories
3 tablespoons oil	375	0	375
3 scallions, finely chopped	30	3	27
2 tablespoons finely diced candied ginger	0	0	0
4 cups hot cooked white rice	800	600	200

Place the oil in a wok. Stir-fry the scallions for about 1 minute. Add the ginger and hot rice and toss together.

Serves 6

Totals	Per Recipe	Per Serving
Calories	1205	201
Blocked Starch Calories	603	101
Remaining Non-Starch Calories	602	100

RICE CREOLE

Ingredients	Calories	Blocked Starch Calories	Remaining Non-Starch Calories
1 cup uncooked long-grain white or brown rice	600	450	150
1 teaspoon salt	0	0	0
1 teaspoon freshly ground black pepper	0	0	0
1 tablespoon minced hot green chili pepper	5	0	5
1 tablespoon whipped butter	70	0	70

Cook the rice according to package directions until tender. Add the remaining ingredients plus 3 cups water. Garnish with tomato wedges and serve with poultry or fish.

Serves 4

Totals	Per Recipe	Per Serving
Calories	675	169
Blocked Starch Calories	450	113
Remaining Non-Starch Calories	225	56

CHINESE FRIED RICE

Ingredients	Calories	Blocked Starch Calories	Remaining Non-Starch Calories
2 tablespoons safflower oil	250	0	250
½ cup finely diced chicken	60	0	60
½ cup sliced mushrooms	20	0	20
4 cups cooked white rice	800	600	200
1 green onion, chopped fine	4	0	4
2 tablespoons soy sauce	8	0	8
1 egg, beaten	80	0	80

Place the oil in a skillet and heat until almost smoking. Cook the chicken in the hot oil for 2 to 3 minutes, add the mushrooms, rice, onion, and the soy sauce. Cook over low heat for about 10 minutes, stirring almost constantly. Add the egg and stir-fry for another 5 minutes.

Serves 6

Totals	Per Recipe	Per Serving
Calories	1222	205
Blocked Starch Calories	600	100
Remaining Non-Starch Calories	622	105

STARCHY VEGETABLES

HONEY MINTED CARROTS

Ingredients	Calories	Blocked Starch Calories	Remaining Non-Starch Calories
6 carrots	210	18	192
1 tablespoon minced fresh mint	0	0	0
1 tablespoon honey	61	0	61

Place the carrots and mint in a saucepan, add water to cover, and cook until carrots are tender. Drain, add the honey, and shake the pan over heat until carrots are coated in honey.

Serves 4

Totals	Per Recipe	Per Serving
Calories	271	68
Blocked Starch Calories	18	5
Remaining Non-Starch Calories	253	63

SUCCOTASH

INGREDIENTS	CALORIES	BLOCKED STARCH CALORIES	REMAINING NON-STARCH CALORIES
1 cup baby green lima beans	220	165	55
1 cup whole-kernel corn	174	131	43
1 tablespoon diced pimiento	0	0	0
Butter-flavored salt	0	0	0

Cook the beans in a small amount of boiling water for about 20 minutes. Add the corn. Bring to a boil, then drain. Add the pimiento and salt.

Serves 4

TOTALS	PER RECIPE	PER SERVING
Calories	394	99
Blocked Starch Calories	296	74
Remaining Non-Starch Calories	98	25

BOSTON'S BEST BAKED BEANS

Ingredients	Calories	Blocked Starch Calories	Remaining Non-Starch Calories
2 cups dried navy beans	1050	788	262
1½ teaspoons salt	0	0	0
1 small minced onion	27	2	25
4 tablespoons molasses	200	0	200
1 teaspoon dry mustard	0	0	0
4 tablespoons chili sauce	14	0	14
1 carrot, diced	35	3	32
4 slices bacon (optional)	180	0	180

Soak the beans overnight in cold water. Preheat the oven to 250°F. Drain the beans, add 2 quarts fresh water, the salt, and the onion and cook until the beans are tender. Drain, and reserve the liquid. Combine the molasses, mustard, chili sauce, carrot, and bacon, if using, with 1 cup of the bean juice and add to the beans. Put bean mixture in a bean pot, cover, and bake in about a 250°F oven for about 3 hours, uncovering for last 30 minutes. If the beans seem too dry at any time, add a little water.

Serves 6

Totals	Per Recipe	Per Serving
Calories	1506	251
Blocked Starch Calories	793	132
Remaining Non-Starch Calories	713	119

FISH

SMOKED SALMON HASH
from the kitchen of chef Philippe Boulot

Ingredients	Calories	Blocked Starch Calories	Remaining Non-Starch Calories
1 pound peeled russet potatoes	440	70	370
1 pound smoked salmon, skinned, boned, and flaked into chunks	750	0	750
4 ounces fresh salmon	150	0	150
¼ red onion, finely diced	8	0	8
1 clove garlic, chopped	0	0	0
1 teaspoon flat-leaf parsley, finely chopped	0	0	0
1 tablespoon horseradish	0	0	0
¼ cup capers, measured, then chopped	4	0	4
2 scallions, finely chopped	4	0	4
1 tablespoon olive oil	125	0	125
8 ounces sour cream	494	0	494

Boil the potatoes until just tender, and allow to cool. Grate the potatoes on the large holes of a box grater; set aside. Mix together both types of salmon, onion, garlic, parsley, horseradish, and capers. The mixture should be moist but not runny. In a large nonstick skillet, or on a seasoned griddle, cook the potatoes in the olive oil until crisp; move to one side of the pan. Add the salmon mixture and cook until heated through. When warm, cut the potatoes into the salmon with a spatula, and continue to cook, allowing the salmon and potatoes to get crisp and brown. When hot, remove to a warm plate and garnish with the scallions and sour cream.

Serves 4

TOTALS	PER RECIPE	PER SERVING
Calories	1970	492
Blocked Starch Calories	70	18
Remaining Non-Starch Calories	1900	475

PESTO-CRUSTED SALMON WITH RED ONION RELISH
from the kitchen of chef Philippe Boulot

INGREDIENTS	CALORIES	BLOCKED STARCH CALORIES	REMAINING NON-STARCH CALORIES
PESTO SALMON			
4 ounces smoked bacon	145	0	145
2 ounces fresh basil	0	0	0
1 ounce toasted pine nuts	50	0	50
6 cloves garlic	5	0	5
2 tablespoons olive oil	250	0	250
Salt and freshly ground pepper	0	0	0
4 salmon fillets (5 ounces each)	938	0	938

Preheat the oven to 350°F. Cut the bacon into chunks, and process in a blender to make a fine paste. Chill. Process the basil, pine nuts, garlic, and oil in a blender or food processor, to make pesto. Combine the pesto with the bacon, and season with salt and pepper. (Test a small amount of the pesto for flavor and texture by frying it in a nonstick pan.) Season the salmon with salt and pepper. Apply some of the pesto to the fleshy side of the fish. Place the fillets crust-side down in hot nonstick pan to sear. Turn the fillets over with a spatula and finish cooking until done.

RELISH

¼ cup olive oil	500	0	500
5 cloves garlic	4	0	4
1 cup finely chopped red onion	54	4	50
3 limes, juiced	60	18	42
1 tablespoon chopped cilantro	0	0	0
1 tablespoon capers	1	0	1

Warm the olive oil in a skillet and add the garlic. Cook the garlic briefly. Sauté the onions in garlic and olive oil slowly, until tender. Stir in the lime juice; let the juice reduce with the onions. Set aside to cool to room temperature. Stir in the cilantro and capers. Serve at room temperature with the pesto-crusted salmon.

Serves 4

TOTALS	PER RECIPE	PER SERVING
Calories	2007	501
Blocked Starch Calories	22	6
Remaining Non-Starch Calories	1985	496

SALMON LOAF

INGREDIENTS	CALORIES	BLOCKED STARCH CALORIES	REMAINING NON-STARCH CALORIES
1 can red or pink salmon	700	0	700
16 soda crackers	280	210	70
1 small onion, diced	27	2	25
½ cup diced celery	10	3	7
1 tablespoon finely chopped green pepper	5	2	3
2 eggs, beaten	150	0	150
1 tablespoon all-purpose flour	25	19	6
Celery salt and freshly ground pepper	0	0	0
Vegetable oil spray for the dish	0	0	0

Preheat the oven to 375°F. Empty the salmon and its liquid into a bowl and remove any large pieces of bone and skin. Crush the crackers and add them, plus the remaining ingredients (except the oil), to the salmon. Mix well and pack into an oiled nonstick baking dish about 4 x 4 x 8 inches. Bake for about 45 minutes, or until lightly browned. Let cool slightly before moving from baking dish to serving platter.

Serves 6

TOTALS	PER RECIPE	PER SERVING
Calories	1197	200
Blocked Starch Calories	236	39
Remaining Non-Starch Calories	961	161

CAJUN COD AND RICE

Ingredients	Calories	Blocked Starch Calories	Remaining Non-Starch Calories
1 pound fresh cod fillets	352	0	352
1 cup sliced scallions (including tops)	54	4	50
1 green pepper, diced	16	0	16
4 fresh tomatoes, chopped (or 1 can)	60	0	60
½ teaspoon dried thyme	0	0	0
½ teaspoon dried oregano	0	0	0
Salt and freshly ground pepper	0	0	0
2 cups cooked brown rice	400	300	100

Preheat the oven to 350°F. Simmer the scallions, green pepper, tomatoes, and seasonings in a saucepan for about 20 minutes. Arrange the cod fillets in a baking dish and pour vegetable sauce over them. Bake for about 20 minutes or until fish begins to flake easily. Serve over hot rice.

Serves 4

Totals	Per Recipe	Per Serving
Calories	882	221
Blocked Starch Calories	304	76
Remaining Non-Starch Calories	578	145

DESSERTS

CHOCOLATE HAZELNUT SHORTCAKE WITH WHITE CHOCOLATE CREAM AND BERRIES
from the kitchen of chef Philippe Boulot

Ingredients	Calories	Blocked Starch Calories	Remaining Non-Starch Calories
SHORTCAKE			
1½ cups all-purpose flour	600	450	150
3 tablespoons granulated sugar, plus more for glaze	135	0	135
1 tablespoon baking powder	0	0	0
¼ teaspoon salt	0	0	0
1 stick cold butter	813	0	813
¼ cup lightly toasted, skinned, and chopped hazelnuts	210	4	206
¼ cup finely chopped semisweet chocolate	201	0	201
⅓ cup whole milk, plus more for glaze	50	0	50
Confectioners' sugar, for dusting	25	0	25

Preheat the oven to 375°F. Sift the dry ingredients together. Cube the butter, and mix with the dry ingredients until the mixture resembles coarse meal. Stir in the hazelnuts and chocolate. Mix in the milk to make a soft dough. You may need to adjust with more or less milk. Turn the dough out onto a lightly floured board and give it 3 to 4 gentle kneads. Pat the dough into a ¾-inch thickness. Using a biscuit cutter or a glass, cut the dough into shortcakes that are about 2½ to 3 inches in diameter. Chill for 30 minutes. Place the shortcakes on a sheet pan and brush the tops with milk and sprinkle with sugar. Bake for 12 to 15 minutes, or until golden brown.

CREAM

2 ounces white chocolate, finely chopped	268	0	268
6 fluid ounces heavy cream	616	0	616

Scald the cream and pour over the chopped white chocolate. Let sit for a few seconds and stir gently, to blend and melt the chocolate. Chill. When the cream is cold, whip it to soft peaks, taking care not to overbeat. To serve, split the cakes, place some berries on each cake, add a dollop of the cream and a few more berries. Top with other half of cake and dust with confectioners' sugar.

Serves 6 to 8

TOTALS	PER RECIPE	PER SERVING (6)	PER SERVING (8)
Calories	2918	486	364
Blocked Starch Calories	454	76	57
Remaining Non-Starch Calories	2464	410	308

ORANGE ALMOND BISCOTTI
from the kitchen of chef Philippe Boulot

INGREDIENTS	CALORIES	BLOCKED STARCH CALORIES	REMAINING NON-STARCH CALORIES
2 cups all-purpose flour	800	600	200
1 teaspoon baking powder	0	0	0
¼ teaspoon salt	0	0	0
4 tablespoons (½ stick) butter	407	0	407
1 cup sugar	720	0	720
2 eggs	150	0	150

Ingredient	Calories	Blocked Starch Calories	Remaining Non-Starch Calories
½ teaspoon vanilla	0	0	0
2 tablespoons grated orange zest	0	0	0
¾ cup I chopped, lightly toasted almonds	630	16	614

Preheat the oven to 350°F. Combine the dry ingredients. Cream the butter and sugar with an electric hand-mixer until light and fluffy, 3 to 4 minutes. Add the eggs one by one, then the vanilla and zest, mixing well after each addition. Sift the dry mix in; add the almonds and mix. On a parchment-lined cookie sheet, roll the dough into rough log shapes the length of the pan, and about 2 inches wide. They will spread out. Bake until golden brown, 25 to 35 minutes. Cool until you can handle them. Lower oven to 300°F. Slice the logs at a slight angle, about ¼ inch wide, with a serrated knife. Put the slices back on the lined sheets and bake until they are dry and lightly browned, about 15 minutes. Then turn the slices over and repeat. Let the cookies cool completely and store in an airtight container.

Makes about 3½ dozen

TOTALS	PER RECIPE	PER SERVING
Calories	2707	65
Blocked Starch Calories	616	15
Remaining Non-Starch Calories	2091	50

RUSTIC BUTTER CAKE
from the kitchen of chef Philippe Boulot

INGREDIENTS	CALORIES	BLOCKED STARCH CALORIES	REMAINING NON-STARCH CALORIES
1½ cups butter	2439	0	2439
1½ cups sugar	1080	0	1080

Grated zest of ½ an orange	0	0	0
6 eggs	450	0	450
1½ tablespoons fresh orange juice	10	0	10
1½ cups all-purpose flour	600	450	150
1½ teaspoons baking powder	0	0	0

Preheat the oven to 350°F. Cream the butter, sugar, and zest with an electric hand-mixer until light and fluffy, 3 to 9 minutes. Add the eggs one by one, beating until fluffy after each egg. Mix in the juice. Sift together the dry ingredients and mix into the batter, scraping the bowl well, and mixing again to incorporate all ingredients. Grease and paper a 9-inch springform pan, and smooth the batter inside. Dust with sugar and a few finely chopped nuts, or a little coconut. Bake for 45 minutes to 1 hour. Unmold when cool. Serve as is, or with fresh berries and stone fruit.

Makes 12 pieces

TOTALS	PER RECIPE	PER SERVING
Calories	4579	382
Blocked Starch Calories	450	38
Remaining Non-Starch Calories	4129	344

HONEY BREAD PUDDING

INGREDIENTS	CALORIES	BLOCKED STARCH CALORIES	REMAINING NON-STARCH CALORIES
2 cups cubed slightly dry bread	440	330	110
Oil spray, for baking dish	0	0	0
2 cups whole milk	300	0	300
2 eggs, beaten	150	0	150
⅓ cup honey	325	0	325
1 teaspoon vanilla	0	0	0

1 cup seedless raisins	460	0	460
1 teaspoon vinegar	0	0	0

Preheat the oven to 375°F. Place the bread cubes in an oil sprayed 8-inch-square baking dish. Mix the remaining ingredients and pour over bread cubes. Place the dish in larger pan and add about 1 inch of water to the larger pan. Bake for about 40 minutes, or until a knife inserted in the center comes out clean.

Serves 8

TOTALS	PER RECIPE	PER SERVING
Calories	1675	209
Blocked Starch Calories	330	41
Remaining Non-Starch Calories	1345	168

OLD-FASHIONED POPPYSEED CAKE
from the kitchen of chef Philippe Boulot

INGREDIENTS	CALORIES	BLOCKED STARCH CALORIES	REMAINING NON-STARCH CALORIES
⅓ cup poppy seeds	244	10	234
¾ cup whole milk	50	0	50
1½ teaspoons vanilla extract	0	0	0
¾ cup butter, room temperature, plus more for pan	1220	0	1220
1½ cups sugar	1080	0	1080
2 cups cake flour, sifted	800	600	200
2½ teaspoons baking powder	0	0	0
¼ teaspoon salt	0	0	0
4 egg whites (½ cup)	68	0	68

Preheat the oven to 375°F. Soak the poppy seeds in milk overnight in the refrigerator. Drain through a fine strainer, reserving the milk; add the vanilla to the milk. Cream the butter with an electric hand-mixer until fluffy, adding the sugar slowly and beating until very light. Mix in the drained poppy seeds. Sift the dry ingredients together. Add to the butter mixture, alternating with the milk and vanilla, beginning and ending with the dry ingredients. In a clean mixing bowl, whip the egg whites with an electric hand-mixer until they are firm, but still soft. Gently fold the whites into the creamed mixture. Place batter in a greased bundt pan and bake for 25 minutes.

Makes 12 pieces

TOTALS	PER RECIPE	PER SERVING
Calories	3462	289
Blocked Starch Calories	610	51
Remaining Non-Starch Calories	2852	238

BRETON BUTTER CAKE
from the kitchen of chef Philippe Boulot

INGREDIENTS	CALORIES	BLOCKED STARCH CALORIES	REMAINING NON-STARCH CALORIES
2 cups all-purpose flour, plus more for pan	800	600	200
1 cup sugar	720	0	720
3 egg yolks	177	0	177
½ pound (2 sticks) butter, softened, plus more for pan	1626	0	1626

Preheat the oven to 350°F. Mix the flour and sugar together in a bowl and make a well. Reserving one egg yolk, put the remaining ingredients in the well. With your hands, mix the wet in with the dry, little by little. Don't overwork. Butter and flour a 9-inch cake pan and fit dough in level. Brush the top with 1 egg yolk mixed with a tiny bit of water. Pull the tines and bake for about 1 hour.

Makes one 9-inch cake, 6 pieces

TOTALS	PER RECIPE	PER SERVING
Calories	3323	554
Blocked Starch Calories	600	100
Remaining Non-Starch Calories	2723	454

ORANGE CHIFFON CAKE
from the kitchen of chef Philippe Boulot

INGREDIENTS	CALORIES	BLOCKED STARCH CALORIES	REMAINING NON-STARCH CALORIES
2¼ cups cake flour, sifted	900	675	225
1½ cups sugar	1080	0	1080
3 teaspoons baking powder	0	0	0
1 teaspoon salt	0	0	0
½ cup vegetable oil	109	0	109
5 egg yolks	295	0	295
¾ cup fresh orange juice	83	0	83
3 tablespoons grated orange zest	0	0	0
7 to 8 egg whites (1 cup)	119	0	119
½ teaspoon cream of tartar	0	0	0

Preheat the oven to 325°F. Sift the flour, sugar, baking powder, and salt into a mixing bowl, and make a well in the center. Put the oil, egg yolks, juice, and zest in the well and mix until smooth and blended. In a clean mixing bowl, whip the egg whites with the cream of tartar with an electric hand-mixer until soft but firm peaks form. Fold the egg whites gently, in 3 portions, into the batter. Be careful not to knock the air out of the mixture. Pour the batter into an ungreased tube pan. Bake for 55 minutes. Lower the temperature to 350°F and bake for 10 to 15 minutes longer. Remove from oven and invert on heavy wine bottle or other object to cool and maintain the cake's structure. When completely cool, go around the edges with a thin spatula or knife, and unmold. Ice as desired or dust with confectioners' sugar. Serve as is, or with fresh fruit.

Makes 10 pieces

TOTALS	PER RECIPE	PER SERVING
Calories	2586	259
Blocked Starch Calories	675	68
Remaining Non-Starch Calories	1911	191

SPICY GINGERBREAD
from the kitchen of chef Philippe Boulot

INGREDIENTS	CALORIES	BLOCKED STARCH CALORIES	REMAINING NON-STARCH CALORIES
½ pound (2 sticks) butter, softened, plus more for pan	1626	0	1626
1 cup sugar	720	0	720
3 eggs	225	0	225
1 cup molasses	872	0	872
2½ cups all-purpose flour, sifted	1000	750	250
1 teaspoon baking soda	0	0	0
2 tablespoons powdered ginger	0	0	0
2 tablespoons ground cinnamon	0	0	0
2 tablespoons ground nutmeg	0	0	0

2 tablespoons ground coriander	0	0	0
2 tablespoons ground cloves	0	0	0

Preheat the oven to 375°F. Cream the butter with an electric mixer until fluffy; add the sugar slowly while mixing. Add the eggs one by one to the butter mixture and beat for 5 minutes. Mix the molasses with ¾ cup water, and beat in. Sift the dry ingredients together and add to the batter. Place in a buttered 13 x 9 x 2-inch pan and bake for 35 to 45 minutes. Serve warm with whipped cream and sautéed pears or apples.

Makes 12 pieces

TOTALS	PER RECIPE	PER SERVING
Calories	4443	370
Blocked Starch Calories	750	63
Remaining Non-Starch Calories	3693	307

BUTTERMILK SCONES
from the kitchen of chef Philippe Boulot

INGREDIENTS	CALORIES	BLOCKED STARCH CALORIES	REMAINING NON-STARCH CALORIES
3¼ cups all-purpose flour	1300	975	325
½ cup sugar, plus more for sprinkling	360	0	360
2½ teaspoons baking powder	0	0	0
½ teaspoon baking soda	0	0	0
½ teaspoon salt	0	0	0
¾ cup cold butter, cut up into pieces	1220	0	1220
1 cup raisins, currants, dried fruit, or berries	200	0	200
1 cup buttermilk	99	0	99
Whole milk for glaze	0	0	0

Preheat the oven to 375°F. Mix the dry ingredients together. Cut in the butter with a pastry cutter or 2 knives until the mixture is crumbly, with only small pieces of butter visible, if any. Toss in the fruit. Mix in the buttermilk, adding more if the dough remains dry and doesn't hold together when squeezed. Divide the dough in half and pat into 2 round balls, then flatten slightly. They should be between 5 and 6 inches in diameter. Cut each into 6 wedges and space them apart on a parchment-lined cookie sheet. Brush the tops with milk and sprinkle generously with sugar. Bake for 20 to 25 minutes, or nicely browned. Don't over-bake.

Serves 12

TOTALS	PER RECIPE	PER SERVING
Calories	3179	265
Blocked Starch Calories	975	81
Remaining Non-Starch Calories	2204	184

BUCKWHEAT CRÊPES BRETONNE
from the kitchen of chef Philippe Boulot

INGREDIENTS	CALORIES	BLOCKED STARCH CALORIES	REMAINING NON-STARCH CALORIES
1 cup all-purpose flour	400	300	100
¾ cup buckwheat flour	300	225	75
¼ teaspoon salt	0	0	0
2 tablespoons sugar	90	0	90
1 egg	75	0	75
2 egg yolks	118	0	118
½ cup whole milk	75	0	75
4 tablespoons butter, melted, plus more for pan	400	0	400

Mix the flours, salt, and sugar in a mixing bowl. Make a well in the flour and add the egg, the yolks, and the milk. With a whisk, mix until the mixture is smooth, with no lumps. Add ½ cup water and butter. Let the batter rest for at least an hour.

Heat a nonstick or cast-iron pan, and when hot, lightly grease with butter, and pour a small amount of batter in the pan, just enough to coat the bottom of the pan. When the crêpe is browned, flip it over and brown the other side. Invert, or slip out onto a large plate, and continue cooking the rest of the batter. Serve with a desired savory filling, or with jam and sugar.

Makes 12

Totals	Per Recipe	Per Serving
Calories	1458	122
Blocked Starch Calories	525	44
Remaining Non-Starch Calories	933	78

RAISIN RICE PUDDING

Ingredients	Calories	Blocked Starch Calories	Remaining Non-Starch Calories
½ cup uncooked rice	300	225	75
4 cups whole milk	600	0	600
½ cup raisins	230	0	230
3 eggs, beaten	240	0	240
½ cup firmly packed brown sugar	400	0	400
1 teaspoon vanilla	0	0	0
¼ teaspoon salt	0	0	0
Cinnamon or nutmeg	0	0	0

Preheat the oven to 350°F. Mix the rice with 2 cups milk. Place the rice mixture in the top of a double boiler and cook over boiling water until the rice is tender. Add the raisins. Combine the eggs, sugar, vanilla, salt, and the remaining 2 cups of milk. Combine the two mixtures and pour into a nonstick baking dish. Sprinkle with cinnamon or nutmeg, or both. Place the baking dish in a pan containing about 2 cups of hot water. Bake for about 45 minutes, or until custard is set.

Serves 6

TOTALS	PER RECIPE	PER SERVING
Calories	1770	295
Blocked Starch Calories	225	38
Remaining Non-Starch Calories	1545	257

ANGEL CAKE

INGREDIENTS	CALORIES	BLOCKED STARCH CALORIES	REMAINING NON-STARCH CALORIES
1 cup cake flour, sifted	400	300	100
1½ cups sugar	540	0	540
12 egg whites (1½ cups)	204	0	204
1½ teaspoons cream of tartar	0	0	0
¼ teaspoon salt	0	0	0
2 teaspoons vanilla	0	0	0
¾ cup sugar	540	0	540

Preheat the oven to 375°F. Sift the flour and ¾ cup sugar 3 or 4 times. Using an electric hand-mixer, beat egg whites with the cream of tartar, salt, and vanilla until soft peaks form but the egg whites are still glossy. Add the remaining ¾ cup of sugar, 2 or 3 tablespoons at a time. Continue to beat until the meringue holds stiff peaks. Sift ¼ of the flour mixture over the egg whites and fold gently. Continue adding flour until all is added. Bake in a

10-inch angel tube pan for 35 to 40 minutes. Invert the pan on a bottle and allow the cake to cool completely before removing from the pan.

Serves 10

Totals	Per Recipe	Per Serving
Calories	1684	168
Blocked Starch Calories	300	30
Remaining Non-Starch Calories	1384	138

ORANGE SPONGE CAKE

Ingredients	Calories	Blocked Starch Calories	Remaining Non-Starch Calories
6 eggs, separated	480	0	480
1 tablespoon grated orange zest	0	0	0
½ cup orange juice	60	0	60
1½ cups sugar	1080	0	1080
1⅓ cups cake flour, sifted	533	400	133
¼ teaspoon salt	0	0	0
1 teaspoon cream of tartar	0	0	0

Preheat the oven to 325°F. Beat the egg yolks until thick, then add the orange zest and orange juice and beat until combined. Gradually beat in 1 cup sugar and the salt. Fold in the flour. In another bowl, beat two egg whites with an electric hand-mixer until foamy, add the cream of tartar, and beat until peaks form. Gradually add the remaining ½ cup of sugar and beat until stiff peaks form. Fold the egg whites into the yolk mixture. Pour into a tube pan and bake for about 55 minutes. Invert pan onto a bottle and cool cake completely before removing from the pan.

Serves 10

Totals	Per Recipe	Per Serving
Calories	2153	215
Blocked Starch Calories	400	40
Remaining Non-Starch Calories	1753	175

FRESH-APPLE PUFF

Ingredients	Calories	Blocked Starch Calories	Remaining Non-Starch Calories
4 fully ripe apples, diced	300	0	300
1 egg white	17	0	17
1 cup apple juice	118	0	118
1 tablespoon honey	61	0	61
1 teaspoon lemon juice	0	0	0
2 tablespoons tapioca	42	32	10
Cinnamon or nutmeg	0	0	0

Wash and core the apples and dice them very fine. Beat the egg white with an electric hand-mixer until it holds soft peaks. Combine the apple juice, honey, and lemon juice with the tapioca in a small saucepan. Stir constantly until the mixture comes to a boil, then cook for 6 to 8 minutes. Add the hot mixture, a small amount at a time, to the egg white, folding it gently. Fold in the diced apples and a touch of cinnamon. Spoon into dessert dishes and chill before serving.

Serves 4

Totals	Per Recipe	Per Serving
Calories	538	135
Blocked Starch Calories	32	8
Remaining Non-Starch Calories	506	127

FLUFFY TAPIOCA PUDDING

Ingredients	Calories	Blocked Starch Calories	Remaining Non-Starch Calories
3 tablespoons minute tapioca	75	56	19
Pinch of salt	0	0	0
1½ tablespoons honey	90	0	90
2 cups whole milk	300	0	300
1 egg, separated	58	0	58
2 tablespoons honey	135	0	135
1 teaspoon vanilla	0	0	0

Mix the tapioca, salt, 2 tablespoons of honey, milk, and beaten egg yolk in a saucepan. Let the mixture stand for 5 minutes. Beat egg white with an electric hand-mixer. Add 1½ tablespoons honey to the egg white and continue beating until it forms soft peaks. Cook the tapioca mixture over medium heat until it comes to a full boil, stirring constantly, 6 to 8 minutes. When pudding is boiling vigorously, gradually add it to the beaten egg white, folding it in quickly just until blended. Stir in the vanilla. The pudding may be served warm or chilled.

Serves 5

Totals	Per Recipe	Per Serving
Calories	675	135
Blocked Starch Calories	56	11
Remaining Non-Starch Calories	619	124

MAIN DISHES

SEAFOOD FETTUCCINE VIN BLANC
from the kitchen of chef Philippe Boulot

Ingredients	Calories	Blocked Starch Calories	Remaining Non-Starch Calories
2 cups white wine	150	0	150
¼ of a "fifth" bottle of dry vermouth	255	0	255
2 ounces shallots, minced	28	1	27
2 cups heavy cream	1642	0	1642
Salt and freshly ground pepper	0	0	0
12 littleneck clams	86	0	86
12 mussels	104	0	104
12 tiger prawns	106	0	106
8 ounces fresh salmon, cut into cubes	354	0	354
1 tablespoon olive oil	125	0	125
2 medium carrots, julienned and blanched	70	6	64
½ bunch scallions, julienned and blanched	30	5	25
1 pound 8 ounces fettuccine pasta, cooked	300	225	75

Combine the wine, vermouth, and shallots in a saucepan, and cook over medium-high heat until reduced to a syrup. Add the cream, bring to a boil, and adjust the seasoning. Chill and reserve. Sauté the seafood in olive oil until the salmon and prawns are just cooked, and the clams and mussels are beginning to open. Add the julienne of carrots and scallions with about 2 cups of the sauce. When hot, toss with freshly cooked pasta and serve.

Serves 4

Totals	Per Recipe	Per Serving
Calories	3245	811
Blocked Starch Calories	237	59
Remaining Non-Starch Calories	3008	752

STUFFED GREEN PEPPERS

Ingredients	Calories	Blocked Starch Calories	Remaining Non-Starch Calories
6 medium green peppers	96	0	96
1 cup uncooked white rice	600	450	150
½ pound ground round (or extra-lean hamburger)	405	0	405
2 tablespoons minced onion	15	1	14
1 tablespoon vegetable oil	120	0	120
1 fourteen-and-a-half-ounce can tomatoes, mashed into small chunks	60	0	60
1 can tomato soup	110	0	110
½ teaspoon dried oregano	0	0	0
Salt and freshly ground pepper	0	0	0
2 ounces grated Cheddar cheese	56	0	56

Preheat the oven to 350°F. Slice the tops from the green peppers, remove fibers and seeds. Boil in salted water for about 10 minutes and drain. Cook the rice according to package directions. Brown the beef and onion in the oil. Mix rice, meat mixture, tomatoes, soup, and oregano together, and salt and pepper to taste. Divide the rice and meat mixture among the peppers, filling to within about ¼ inch of the tops. Place the peppers in a baking dish with a cover. Pour a cup of water around them. Cover and bake for 1 hour. Uncover, sprinkle the grated cheese on top of the peppers, and leave in oven until cheese is melted and starts to brown.

Serves 6

TOTALS	PER RECIPE	PER SERVING
Calories	1462	244
Blocked Starch Calories	451	75
Remaining Non-Starch Calories	1011	169

WHOLE WHEAT COUSCOUS WITH CECI AND GOLDEN RAISINS
from the kitchen of chef Philippe Boulot

INGREDIENTS	CALORIES	BLOCKED STARCH CALORIES	REMAINING NON-STARCH CALORIES
14 ounces chicken stock	30	0	30
1 tablespoon olive oil	125	0	125
1 cup whole wheat couscous	160	40	120
⅓ cup canned ceci (chickpeas), rinsed and drained	87	14	73
Small handful of raisins	200	0	200
Small sprig fresh thyme	0	0	0

Bring the stock to a boil. Warm the olive oil in a small saucepan and add the couscous, stirring to coat the grains. Pour the stock over the grains and quickly drop in the ceci, raisins, and thyme. Cover, and turn off the burner. Let stand for about 8 minutes. Uncover and fluff the couscous. Recover and let stand for a few more minutes. Serve with steamed vegetables. A pinch of curry can be added with the thyme, if desired.

Serves 4

TOTALS	PER RECIPE	PER SERVING
Calories	623	156
Blocked Starch Calories	54	14
Remaining Non-Starch Calories	569	142

TAMALE PIE

INGREDIENTS	CALORIES	BLOCKED STARCH CALORIES	REMAINING NON-STARCH CALORIES
1 chopped onion	35	3	32
1 chopped green pepper	16	0	16
1 pound ground round (or extra-lean hamburger)	810	0	810
1 green chili, chopped	5	0	5
2 eight-ounce cans seasoned tomato sauce	680	0	680
1 twelve-ounce can whole-kernel corn, drained	174	131	43
1 clove garlic, minced	0	0	0
1 tablespoon sugar	45	0	45
1 teaspoon salt	0	0	0
3 teaspoons chili powder	0	0	0
1 cup Cheddar cheese	480	0	480
CORNMEAL TOP			
¾ cup yellow cornmeal	285	214	71
½ teaspoon salt	0	0	0
1 tablespoon whipped butter	70	0	70

Preheat the oven to 350°F. Cook the onions and peppers in 1 tablespoon of hot fat in a large skillet until tender, then add the meat, and brown. Add all other ingredients except the cheese and topping mix. Cook slowly for about 25 minutes. Add the cheese and stir until melted. Pour in a baking dish. Make the cornmeal topping: Place 2 cups cold water in a saucepan and stir in the cornmeal and salt. Simmer, stirring until thick. Add butter, and mix well. Spoon cornmeal top over meat mixture. Bake for about 1 hour.

Serves 10

Totals	Per Recipe	Per Serving
Calories	2600	260
Blocked Starch Calories	348	35
Remaining Non-Starch Calories	2252	225

ITALIAN MACARONI AND TOMATOES

Ingredients	Calories	Blocked Starch Calories	Remaining Non-Starch Calories
1 eight-ounce package elbow macaroni	840	630	210
2 tablespoons whipped butter, plus more for dish	140	0	140
2 tablespoons all-purpose flour	50	38	12
2 cups whole milk	300	0	300
1 cup grated Cheddar cheese	450	0	450
2 cups soft breadcrumbs	440	330	110
3 medium tomatoes, sliced	75	0	75
Salt and freshly ground pepper	0	0	0
½ teaspoon dried dill weed	0	0	0
½ teaspoon dried basil	0	0	0

Preheat the oven to 350°F. Cook the macaroni in salted water according to package directions and drain. Make a white sauce by melting the butter, stirring in the flour, then the milk, and cooking until it thickens. Add ¾ cup of cheese to the white sauce. Butter a casserole dish. Place one-half of the macaroni in the casserole, add half the breadcrumbs and tomatoes, and pour half the sauce over that. Sprinkle with salt, pepper, ¼ teaspoon dill weed, and ¼ teaspoon basil. Then repeat with the remaining macaroni, breadcrumbs, and tomatoes, and sprinkle the top with the remaining ¼ cup of cheese. Bake for 45 to 50 minutes.

Serves 8

TOTALS	PER RECIPE	PER SERVING
Calories	2295	230
Blocked Starch Calories	998	100
Remaining Non-Starch Calories	1297	130

CHICKEN ARTICHOKE HASH WITH POACHED EGGS AND TARRAGON CRÈME FRAÎCHE
from the kitchen of chef Philippe Boulot

INGREDIENTS	CALORIES	BLOCKED STARCH CALORIES	REMAINING NON-STARCH CALORIES
1 small yellow onion, julienned and caramelized	27	2	25
1 tablespoon olive oil	125	0	125
¼ cup lemon juice	13	3	10
¼ cup chicken stock	8	0	8
¼ cup extra-virgin olive oil	477	0	477
1 garlic glove	0	0	0
1 small bunch tarragon, leaves picked, chopped	14	0	14
Salt and freshly ground pepper			
1 pound baby artichokes	120	24	96
1 red pepper, diced	20	3	17
1 green pepper, diced	20	8	12
1 pound boneless, skinless chicken thighs, roasted, diced	300	0	300
1 pound Yukon gold potatoes, roasted, diced	220	35	185
4 ounces sour cream	247	0	247
¼ cup heavy cream	205	0	205

Butter for pan	25	0	25
4 eggs	300	0	300

Start by caramelizing the onion; cook the onion slowly in olive oil, stirring it as it browns. When it is golden, and starts to stick to the pan, remove and reserve to the side. In a small saucepan, combine the lemon juice, chicken stock, and oil. Bring to a boil and add garlic, a pinch of tarragon, salt, and pepper. Trim the artichokes, pare the bases, and cut in half. If the artichoke heart is tough and spiky, scoop it out with a teaspoon. Cook the artichokes in chicken stock mixture, simmering until tender. Remove and cool. Combine the cooled artichokes, diced peppers, onions, chicken, potatoes, and about half of the tarragon. Season and mix. Make the tarragon cream: Combine the sour cream, cream, and tarragon. Season to taste. Heat some butter in a cast-iron skillet or a griddle and cook the hash until crispy and hot. Meanwhile, poach the eggs to desired doneness. Divide the hash among 4 plates. Top each serving with a poached egg and drizzle the tarragon cream over the top.

Serves 4

TOTALS	PER RECIPE	PER SERVING
Calories	2121	530
Blocked Starch Calories	75	19
Remaining Non-Starch Calories	2046	571

GRILLED POLENTA WITH PIPERADE BASQUAISE
from the kitchen of chef Philippe Boulot

INGREDIENTS	CALORIES	BLOCKED STARCH CALORIES	REMAINING NON-STARCH CALORIES
5 cups chicken stock	75	0	75
1 teaspoon salt	0	0	0

1½ cups cornmeal	266	200	66
½ cup grated Parmesan cheese	227	0	227
¾ cup Mascarpone cheese	480	0	480
Olive oil, for pan	0	0	0

Bring the stock to a boil; add salt and whisk in the cornmeal. Cook, stirring, for 20 minutes until polenta is as thick as mashed potatoes. Add the Parmesan and stir in the Mascarpone, seasoning to taste. Pour into a shallow, oiled pan. Chill, and let set until firm. Cut into triangles. Either brush with olive oil and grill, or dredge in flour and sauté in olive oil until crispy. Serve with a spoonful of piperade.

PIPERADE BASQUAISE

2 red peppers	40	6	34
2 yellow peppers	40	12	28
2 orange peppers	40	12	28
1 onion	35	3	32
1 tablespoon olive oil	125	0	125
2 large ripe tomatoes	52	0	52
Handful Niçoise olives, pitted	45	0	45
Balsamic vinegar	0	0	0

Julienne the peppers, onion, and tomatoes. Sauté all together until soft and cooked. Add the olives and season to taste with balsamic vinegar. Serve hot or cold with the polenta.

Serves 4

TOTALS	PER RECIPE	PER SERVING
Calories	1425	556
Blocked Starch Calories	233	58
Remaining Non-Starch Calories	1192	298

CHICKEN WITH CHANTERELLE
CREAM SAUCE AND FETTUCCINE
from the kitchen of chef Philippe Boulot

INGREDIENTS	CALORIES	BLOCKED STARCH CALORIES	REMAINING NON-STARCH CALORIES
4 boneless, skinless chicken breasts	336	0	336
1 tablespoon olive oil	125	0	125
2 shallots, minced	28	1	27
1 pound chanterelle mushrooms, cleaned	60	9	51
3 tablespoons white vermouth	25	0	25
1 cup cream	699	0	699
12 ounces fettuccine pasta, cooked	150	113	37
Salt and freshly ground pepper	0	0	0
Fresh snipped chives	0	0	0

Julienne the chicken and brown the meat in batches in the olive oil. Remove the chicken to a plate and keep covered. Add the shallots and mushrooms to the pan and cook. Add the vermouth and let it reduce, then add the cream. Put the chicken back into the pan and let it warm up in the sauce. Season to taste. Add the freshly cooked pasta and toss gently. Sprinkle chives over the top.

Serves 4

TOTALS	PER RECIPE	PER SERVING
Calories	1423	355
Blocked Starch Calories	123	31
Remaining Non-Starch Calories	1300	325

PAPPARDELLE WITH DUCK CONFIT
from the kitchen of chef Philippe Boulot

INGREDIENTS	CALORIES	BLOCKED STARCH CALORIES	REMAINING NON-STARCH CALORIES
Salt and freshly ground pepper	0	0	0
4 duck legs	1287	0	1287
1 medium carrot, diced	35	3	32
1 onion, diced	35	3	32
1 stalk celery, diced	10	3	7
1 tablespoon all-purpose flour	25	19	6
2 tablespoons tomato paste	27	0	27
12 ounces pappardelle pasta, cooked	150	113	37

Salt and pepper the duck legs. Brown them evenly in a medium saucepan. Remove the legs to a plate and add the carrot, onion, and celery; sauté. Add the flour, stirring to make a soft, semifluid paste. Add the tomato paste and let cook a few minutes on low heat. Put the duck legs back in the pot and add just enough water to cover the duck. Simmer until the meat is tender and falling from the bones, checking the seasoning halfway through. Remove the meat from the bones and shred, letting the liquid reduce to a light sauce consistency. Add the meat back to the liquid and toss this with freshly cooked pappardelle.

Serves 4

TOTALS	PER RECIPE	PER SERVING
Calories	1569	392
Blocked Starch Calories	141	35
Remaining Non-Starch Calories	1428	357

DEEP DISH PIZZA

Ingredients	Calories	Blocked Starch Calories	Remaining Non-Starch Calories
Crust			
1 package dry yeast	0	0	0
1 tablespoon honey	65	0	65
1 tablespoon oil	120	0	120
1 teaspoon salt	0	0	0
2½ cups all-purpose flour	1000	750	250
Sauce			
2 onions, diced	70	6	64
1 clove of garlic	0	0	0
1 tablespoon vegetable oil	120	0	120
1 sixteen-ounce can diced tomatoes	120	0	120
1 six-ounce can tomato paste	138	0	138
1 tablespoon oregano	0	0	0
1 tablespoon basil	0	0	0
1 cup chopped mushrooms	40	0	40
1 cup chopped green peppers	20	0	20
1 cup grated mozzarella cheese	425	0	425

Preheat the oven to 400°F. Sauté the onions and garlic in oil. Add the tomatoes, tomato paste, oregano, and basil and bring to a boil. Add the mushrooms and green pepper. Simmer. For the crust, dissolve the yeast in water, add the honey, oil, and salt, and stir together. Combine this with the flour in a large bowl. Knead the mixture until it's smooth, then roll it out on a floured surface, and trim it to fit a rectangular baking dish. Bake the crust for about 15 minutes, or until lightly browned. Remove the crust from the oven, pour on the sauce, and top with the cheese. Bake for 5 more minutes or until the cheese is melted and slightly brown.

Serves 8

TOTALS	PER RECIPE	PER SERVING
Calories	2118	265
Blocked Starch Calories	756	95
Remaining Non-Starch Calories	1362	170

LAZY DAY SPAGHETTI

INGREDIENTS	CALORIES	BLOCKED STARCH CALORIES	REMAINING NON-STARCH CALORIES
½ pound ground round (or extra-lean hamburger)	405	0	405
1 green pepper, minced	16	0	16
1 onion, minced	35	3	32
1 cup sliced mushrooms	40	0	40
8-ounce package of spaghetti, cooked	100	75	25
2 teaspoons salt	0	0	0
1 teaspoon sugar	15	0	15
3 cups of cooked, canned tomatoes	180	0	180

Preheat the oven to 350°F. Brown the ground round in a skillet. Add the green pepper, onion, and mushrooms. Add the beef to the cooked, drained spaghetti. Add the salt, sugar, and tomatoes and pour into buttered 2-quart casserole dish, sprayed with vegetable oil. Bake for about 30 minutes.

Serves 8

TOTALS	PER RECIPE	PER SERVING
Calories	791	99
Blocked Starch Calories	78	10
Remaining Non-Starch Calories	713	89

CHICKEN PAPRIKA

INGREDIENTS	CALORIES	BLOCKED STARCH CALORIES	REMAINING NON-STARCH CALORIES
4 pieces chicken, breasts or thighs	960	0	960
½ cup whole milk	75	0	75
Salt and freshly ground pepper			
Paprika	0	0	0
1 cup breadcrumbs	330	248	82
Lemon-flavored salt	0	0	0

Preheat the oven to 350°F. Roll the chicken pieces in the milk. Sprinkle with salt and pepper, and a generous amount of paprika. Then roll in the breadcrumbs until well coated. Place in a nonstick baking pan. Cover with foil, and bake for about 30 minutes. Uncover and bake until crispy.

Serves 4

TOTALS	PER RECIPE	PER SERVING
Calories	1365	341
Blocked Starch Calories	248	62
Remaining Non-Starch Calories	1117	279

STIR-FRIED RICE AND VEGETABLES

Ingredients	Calories	Blocked Starch Calories	Remaining Non-Starch Calories
2 beef bouillon cubes	10	0	10
Salt			
1 cup uncooked long-grain rice	600	450	150
1 cup sliced carrots	70	6	64
1 cup sliced celery	20	6	14
½ cup chopped green pepper	10	0	10
¼ cup sliced onions	15	2	13
1 cup snow-pea pods	70	0	70

Bring 3 cups of water to a boil. Add a pinch of salt, the bouillon cubes, and rice. Cook until the rice is tender. Drain if necessary, and keep hot.

Arrange the cooked rice on a large platter. Make a hollow center so it will hold the cooked vegetables. Mix the vegetables, lightly stir-fry all of them together with a touch of olive oil, and add them to the hollow center of the rice. Garnish with parsley and lemon wedges. Serve with soy sauce.

Serves 6

Totals	Per Recipe	Per Serving
Calories	795	133
Blocked Starch Calories	464	77
Remaining Non-Starch Calories	331	56

BUTTERY MACARONI AND CHEESE

INGREDIENTS	CALORIES	BLOCKED STARCH CALORIES	REMAINING NON-STARCH CALORIES
1 seven- or eight-ounce package elbow macaroni	840	630	210
½ teaspoon salt	0	0	0
1 tablespoon butter	100	0	100
1 tablespoon all-purpose flour	25	19	6
2 cups 2% milk	242	0	242
1 cup grated Cheddar cheese	450	0	450
Freshly ground pepper	0	0	0

Preheat the oven to 375°F. Boil macaroni in salted water until barely tender, and drain. Make a white sauce by melting the butter in small saucepan. Add the flour to the butter and mix well; cook until paste no longer tastes like flour before gradually adding the milk. Stir constantly until thickened. Add ¾ cup of cheese, mix into white sauce, and season with salt and pepper to taste. Combine the sauce with the macaroni in a casserole or baking dish, and sprinkle the remaining ¼ cup of cheese on top. Bake for about 45 minutes.

Serves 8

TOTALS	PER RECIPE	PER SERVING
Calories	1657	207
Blocked Starch Calories	649	81
Remaining Non-Starch Calories	1008	126

HUNTINGTON CHICKEN

Ingredients	Calories	Blocked Starch Calories	Remaining Non-Starch Calories
1 cup chopped cooked chicken	120	0	120
1 cup sliced mushrooms	40	0	40
1 cup sliced water chestnuts	120	0	120
1 cup chopped spinach	50	0	50
1 onion, chopped	35	3	32
1 tablespoon soy sauce	8	0	8
2 cups cooked noodles	400	300	100
1 can mushroom soup	195	0	195

Preheat the olive oil to 375°F. Mix all the ingredients and pour into a nonstick baking dish. Cover and bake for about 35 minutes. Uncover and bake for 10 more minutes.

Serves 4

Totals	Per Recipe	Per Serving
Calories	968	242
Blocked Starch Calories	303	76
Remaining Non-Starch Calories	665	166

TAHITIAN CHICKEN

Ingredients	Calories	Blocked Starch Calories	Remaining Non-Starch Calories
1 cup cooked rice	200	150	50
3 large chicken breasts, skinned, split, and boned	720	0	720

1 egg, beaten	75	0	75
2 tablespoons all-purpose flour	90	68	22
2 tablespoons safflower or olive oil	240	0	240
1 four-ounce can pineapple chunks, unsweetened	380	0	380
1⅓ tablespoons honey	86	0	86
3 tablespoons vinegar	2	0	2
4 tablespoons soy sauce	32	0	32
½ teaspoon ground ginger or grated ginger root	0	0	0
1 cup sliced celery	20	6	14
1 large green pepper, cut into chunks	16	0	16
4 tablespoons cornstarch	120	90	30

Cook the rice according to package instructions. Dip the chicken in beaten egg and then flour, and brown in the 2 tablespoons oil. Drain on paper towels and reserve pan drippings. Drain the pineapple, reserving the juice, and add enough water to the juice to make 2 cups. Add the juice, honey, vinegar, soy sauce, and ginger to the pan drippings. Heat. Add the celery and green pepper. Cook until vegetables are barely tender. Mix the cornstarch and 4 tablespoons water and use as necessary to thicken vegetable mix. Add chicken and pineapple chunks and simmer 20 minutes. Serve on hot rice.

Serves 6

TOTALS	PER RECIPE	PER SERVING	
Calories	1981	330	
Blocked Starch Calories	314	52	
Remaining Non-Starch Calories	1667	278	

CHICKEN AND RICE CASSEROLE

Ingredients	Calories	Blocked Starch Calories	Remaining Non-Starch Calories
1 six-ounce package long-grain and wild rice mix	450	338	112
3 large chicken breasts, boned and halved	720	0	720
Salt and freshly ground pepper	0	0	0
2 tablespoons whipped butter	140	0	140
1 twelve- to fourteen-ounce can chicken broth	30	0	30
½ cup sliced celery	10	3	7
1 three-ounce can sliced mushrooms, or ½ cup sliced fresh mushrooms	20	0	20
½ teaspoon curry powder	0	0	0

Preheat the oven to 350°F. Cook the rice according to package instructions. Season the chicken breasts with salt and pepper. Heat the butter in a skillet, and brown the chicken. Place the rice in a casserole dish and top with the browned chicken breast. Add the broth to the skillet, bring to a boil, and add the celery, mushrooms, and curry powder. Pour the broth mixture over the chicken. Cover and bake for about 30 minutes. Uncover and, if rice seems too dry, add about ½ cup water and bake 15 to 20 minutes longer.

Serves 6

Totals	Per Recipe	Per Serving
Calories	1370	228
Blocked Starch Calories	341	56
Remaining Non-Starch Calories	1029	172

ESCALLOPED OYSTERS

Ingredients	Calories	Blocked Starch Calories	Remaining Non-Starch Calories
4 tablespoons whipped butter, melted	400	0	400
1½ cups cracker crumbs	495	371	124
5 tablespoons whole milk	45	0	45
1 pint oysters, with liquid	360	0	360

Preheat the oven to 350°F. Mix the butter with the cracker crumbs. Place a layer of crumbs in the bottom of baking dish, then add a layer of oysters. Make another layer of crumbs, another of oysters, and top with more crumbs. Cover and bake for 30 minutes. Uncover and bake until crumbs are golden brown.

Serves 6

Totals	Per Recipe	Per Serving
Calories	1300	217
Blocked Starch Calories	371	62
Remaining Non-Starch Calories	929	155

SICILIAN MEATBALLS

Ingredients	Calories	Blocked Starch Calories	Remaining Non-Starch Calories
1 pound ground round (or extra-lean hamburger)	810	0	810
½ cup uncooked white rice	300	225	75
2 tablespoons grated onion	15	1	14

1 teaspoon salt	0	0	0
¼ teaspoon freshly ground pepper	0	0	0
½ teaspoon dried oregano	0	0	0
½ teaspoon dried thyme	0	0	0
1 can tomato soup	30	0	30

Preheat the oven to 375°F. Mix the ground beef, rice, onion, salt, pepper, and herbs. Shape into 12 small meatballs. In a covered baking dish, mix the soup and 1 can of water. Place the meatballs and the tomato mixture in a baking dish and bake, covered, for 1 hour.

Serves 6

TOTALS	PER RECIPE	PER SERVING
Calories	1155	193
Blocked Starch Calories	226	38
Remaining Non-Starch Calories	929	155

SPAGHETTI PIE

INGREDIENTS	CALORIES	BLOCKED STARCH CALORIES	REMAINING NON-STARCH CALORIES
6 ounces uncooked spaghetti	630	473	157
2 tablespoons whipped butter, plus more for pan	140	0	140
2 tablespoons grated Parmesan cheese	40	0	40
2 eggs, beaten	150	0	150
1 cup cottage cheese	200	0	200
½ cup chopped onion	27	2	25
½ cup diced celery	10	3	7
2 cups meatless spaghetti sauce	280	210	70

1 teaspoon sugar	15	0	15
1 teaspoon oregano	0	0	0
½ cup shredded mozzarella cheese	212	0	212

Preheat the oven to 350°F. Cook the spaghetti according to package instructions, and drain. Stir in the butter, Parmesan cheese, and eggs. Use the spaghetti to form a crust in a buttered 10-inch pie pan or plate. Spread the cottage cheese over the bottom of the crust. Mix and heat all other ingredients, except the mozzarella, in a saucepan. Pour the spaghetti sauce over the cottage cheese. Bake for about 20 minutes. Sprinkle the mozzarella on top and bake another 5 minutes or until the cheese is melted and bubbly.

Serves 6

TOTALS	PER RECIPE	PER SERVING
Calories	1704	284
Blocked Starch Calories	688	115
Remaining Non-Starch Calories	1016	169

BEEF CHOP SUEY

INGREDIENTS	CALORIES	BLOCKED STARCH CALORIES	REMAINING NON-STARCH CALORIES
1 pound lean beef, sliced into strips about ⅟₁₆ inch thick and 2 inches long	640	0	640
Vegetable oil spray for browning beef	0	0	0
1 onion, chopped	35	3	32
2 cups sliced celery	40	12	28
1 cup sliced mushrooms	40	0	40
1 can bean sprouts, drained, or 2 cups fresh	40	0	40

1 green pepper, cut in thin strips	16	0	16
Salt and freshly ground pepper	0	0	0
3 tablespoons soy sauce	24	0	24
2 tablespoons cornstarch	60	45	15
6 to 8 cups cooked white rice	1200	900	300

Brown the beef strips in a small amount of vegetable oil spray in a hot skillet. Add water, cover, and simmer for about 15 minutes. Add the onion, celery, mushrooms, bean sprouts, green pepper, salt, and pepper. Cook 5 minutes more. Make a paste out of the soy sauce and cornstarch, and use to thicken the chop suey. Serve over the cooked rice.

Serves 6–8

TOTALS	PER RECIPE	PER SERVING (6)	PER SERVING (8)
Calories	2095	349	262
Blocked Starch Calories	960	160	120
Remaining Non-Starch Calories	1135	189	142

SPAGHETTINI WITH SAUCE VERDANT

INGREDIENTS	CALORIES	BLOCKED STARCH CALORIES	REMAINING NON-STARCH CALORIES
8 ounces spaghettini or vermicelli	840	630	210
2 tablespoons whole basil	0	0	0
2 tablespoons parsley flakes	0	0	0
2 tablespoons minced celery leaves	0	0	0
1 teaspoon minced onion	0	0	0
1 eight-ounce package cream cheese, softened	800	0	800

⅓ cup grated Parmesan cheese	106	0	106
1 clove garlic, minced	0	0	0
½ teaspoon freshly ground pepper	0	0	0
Parsley sprigs	0	0	0

Cook the spaghettini in salted, boiling water until barely tender. Drain and keep warm. Place the remaining ingredients in a blender and barely mix. Place the spaghettini in a serving bowl. Stir ⅔ cup hot water into the sauce, and pile sauce atop spaghettini. Garnish with parsley sprigs. Serve with a crisp green salad.

Serves 8

TOTALS	PER RECIPE	PER SERVING
Calories	1746	218
Blocked Starch Calories	630	79
Remaining Non-Starch Calories	1116	139

VEAL STEW WITH PARSLEY DUMPLINGS

INGREDIENTS	CALORIES	BLOCKED STARCH CALORIES	REMAINING NON-STARCH CALORIES
1 pound cubed veal stew meat	640	0	640
1 teaspoon salt	0	0	0
½ teaspoon freshly ground pepper	0	0	0
1 bay leaf	0	0	0
3 potatoes, cubed	360	270	90
3 carrots, cubed	105	9	96
1 cup fresh peas	165	124	41
1 onion, diced	35	3	32
1 tablespoon all-purpose flour	25	19	6

Brown the veal in olive oil in a large Dutch oven, or pot. When browned, add 3 cups water, the salt, pepper, and bay leaf. Cover pan and simmer until meat is tender. Remove the bay leaf and add the vegetables. Cover and simmer until the vegetables are tender. Mix the flour with a little water to make a paste. Add to the stew to thicken. Drop dumplings on top by the teaspoonful. Cover and simmer 10 minutes more.

DUMPLINGS

2 cups all-purpose flour	800	600	200
2 teaspoons baking powder	0	0	0
1 teaspoon salt	0	0	0
1 cup whole milk	150	0	150
2 tablespoons minced fresh parsley	0	0	0

Mix the flour, baking powder, and salt. Add the milk and parsley, and stir only until well mixed.

Serves 6

TOTALS	PER RECIPE	PER SERVING
Calories	2296	383
Blocked Starch Calories	1037	173
Remaining Non-Starch Calories	1259	210

TURKEY SOUFFLÉ

INGREDIENTS	CALORIES	BLOCKED STARCH CALORIES	REMAINING NON-STARCH CALORIES
16 slices bread (crusts removed)	1600	1200	400
8 thin slices turkey	965	0	965
8 slices American cheese	840	0	840

8 eggs	600	0	600
2 teaspoons dry mustard	0	0	0
3 cups whole milk	450	0	450
2 tablespoons whipped butter	200	0	200
1 teaspoon salt	0	0	0
3 cups cornflakes	300	225	75

Arrange half of the bread slices in a large baking pan. Place a slice of turkey and cheese on each slice of bread, then top with another slice of bread. Beat the eggs, add the remaining ingredients, except the cornflakes, and pour over the bread, cheese, and turkey. Refrigerate for 12 hours. Preheat the oven to 325°F. Crush the cornflakes and sprinkle them over the top. Bake for about 1 hour.

Serves 16

TOTALS	PER RECIPE	PER SERVING
Calories	4955	310
Blocked Starch Calories	1425	89
Remaining Non-Starch Calories	3530	221

CHICKEN POTATO PUFF

INGREDIENTS	CALORIES	BLOCKED STARCH CALORIES	REMAINING NON-STARCH CALORIES
4 large potatoes	580	435	145
2 cups chicken broth	30	0	30
1 tablespoon chopped onion	8	0	8
½ cup diced celery	10	3	7
1 chicken breast, broiled and diced	120	0	120
1 tablespoon cornstarch	30	23	7

Butter-flavored salt	0	0	0
Freshly ground pepper	0	0	0
1 tablespoon chopped fresh parsley	0	0	0

Preheat the oven to 375°F. Peel the potatoes and cut into 1-inch-thick slices. Place 1 cup of the chicken broth in a 2-quart saucepan, bring to a boil, add the potatoes, and cook until tender. While potatoes are cooking, cook the onions and celery in the remaining cup of broth in a saucepan. Broil the chicken breast, or pan-fry it, if preferred, and dice into small chunks. When celery is tender, add the chicken. Mix the cornstarch with 2 tablespoons of water to make a paste, and use it to thicken the celery and chicken mixture. Pour this mixture into a baking dish. When the potatoes are tender, drain off all but ¼ cup of the broth. Mash the potatoes and whip until fluffy. Add the salt, pepper, and chopped parsley. Spoon the whipped potatoes over the chicken mixture. Bake for 25 to 35 minutes, or until the potatoes are slightly browned.

Serves 4

TOTALS	PER RECIPE	PER SERVING
Calories	778	195
Blocked Starch Calories	461	115
Remaining Non-Starch Calories	317	79

MEXICALI CORNBREAD SUPPER

INGREDIENTS	CALORIES	BLOCKED STARCH CALORIES	REMAINING NON-STARCH CALORIES
½ pound ground round (or extra-lean hamburger)	405	0	405
1¼ cups stone-ground yellow cornmeal	475	356	119
¼ teaspoon baking soda	0	0	0
2 eggs, beaten	150	0	150

1 cup 2% milk	121	0	121
Celery salt	0	0	0
1 can cream-style corn	174	131	43
2 jalapeño peppers, chopped fine	10	0	10
1 onion, chopped	35	3	32
Freshly ground pepper	0	0	0

Preheat the oven to 375°F. Select a heavy, large skillet, preferably cast-iron. Brown the beef in the skillet, then lift it out and drain off most of the fat. Mix 1 cup cornmeal and the baking soda in a large bowl; add the eggs, milk, celery salt, and corn. Mix well. Stir the remaining ¼ cup cornmeal with the fat remaining in the skillet, and brown. Spoon half the cornbread mixture into the skillet, add half the browned beef, and sprinkle with the jalapeño pepper, ground pepper, and onion. Repeat layers. Bake for 50 to 60 minutes.

Serves 8

Totals	Per Recipe	Per Serving
Calories	1370	171
Blocked Starch Calories	490	61
Remaining Non-Starch Calories	880	110

PRUSSIAN CABBAGE ROLLS

Ingredients	Calories	Blocked Starch Calories	Remaining Non-Starch Calories
6 large cabbage leaves	8	1	7
1 cup uncooked white rice	600	450	150
½ pound ground round (or extra-lean hamburger)	405	0	405
1 onion, chopped	35	3	32
1 tablespoon whipped butter	70	0	70

Ingredient	Calories	Blocked Starch Calories	Remaining Non-Starch Calories
Salt and freshly ground pepper	0	0	0
1 tablespoon lemon juice	0	0	0
1 can tomato soup	110	0	110
½ cup chopped celery	10	3	7
1 teaspoon sugar	15	0	15
1 teaspoon minced fresh parsley	0	0	0
½ teaspoon marjoram	0	0	0

Preheat the oven to 350°F. Drop the cabbage leaves in boiling, salted water for about 2 minutes, to soften. Cook the rice and drain. Brown the ground round and onion in butter. Combine the meat mixture with the rice, and season with salt and pepper. Make a sauce of the lemon juice, soup, 1 cup water, the celery, sugar, parsley, and marjoram. Divide the meat mixture among the cabbage leaves. Roll them up and fasten with toothpicks. Place in a baking dish with a cover. Pour the sauce over them and bake for about 1½ hours. Uncover the last 20 minutes to let the sauce thicken.

Serves 6

TOTALS	PER RECIPE	PER SERVING
Calories	1253	209
Blocked Starch Calories	457	76
Remaining Non-Starch Calories	796	133

CHICKEN OR TURKEY NOODLE CASSEROLE

INGREDIENTS	CALORIES	BLOCKED STARCH CALORIES	REMAINING NON-STARCH CALORIES
1 cup cooked diced chicken or turkey	120	0	120
4 cups cooked noodles	800	600	200
½ cup sliced celery	10	3	7

1 tablespoon chopped onion	8	0	8
1 can cream of mushroom soup	130	0	130
Celery salt	0	0	0
Freshly ground pepper	0	0	0
½ cup breadcrumbs	165	124	41

Preheat the oven to 350°F. Broil or pan-fry the chicken or turkey, and dice it into small chunks. Mix the first 5 ingredients plus 1 soup can of water. Add salt and pepper to taste. Spoon the mixture into a buttered casserole dish and top with breadcrumbs. Cover and bake for 30 minutes. Uncover and bake until the breadcrumbs are browned.

Serves 4

TOTALS	PER RECIPE	PER SERVING
Calories	1233	308
Blocked Starch Calories	727	182
Remaining Non-Starch Calories	506	126

QUICK SHRIMP AND RICE

INGREDIENTS	CALORIES	BLOCKED STARCH CALORIES	REMAINING NON-STARCH CALORIES
2 slices bacon	90	0	90
1 small onion, diced	27	2	25
1 fourteen-and-a-half-ounce can tomatoes	60	0	60
1 cup Minute Rice, uncooked	600	450	150
1 pound shrimp, peeled	480	0	480
¼ teaspoon mace	0	0	0
Salt	0	0	0

Tomato wedges	20	0	20
Parsley snips	0	0	0
Snipped fresh chives	0	0	0

Cube the bacon and fry it until crisp. Drain grease. In the same pan, brown the onion in olive oil. Add the tomatoes and cook 5 minutes. Add the rice and shrimp and cook until rice is done. Add the mace and salt. Garnish with fresh tomato wedges, parsley sprigs, and snipped chives.

Serves 4

TOTALS	PER RECIPE	PER SERVING
Calories	1277	319
Blocked Starch Calories	452	113
Remaining Non-Starch Calories	825	206

STUFFED CUBE STEAKS

INGREDIENTS	CALORIES	BLOCKED STARCH CALORIES	REMAINING NON-STARCH CALORIES
4 cube steaks (¼ pound each)	960	0	960
1 cup bread cubes	220	165	55
1 small onion, chopped	27	2	25
½ cup diced celery	10	3	7
1 teaspoon dried sage	0	0	0
1½ cups beef bouillon	10	0	10
Salt and freshly ground pepper	0	0	0
Cornstarch	0	0	0

Preheat the oven to 350°F. Combine the bread cubes, onion, celery, sage, and ½ cup of bouillon. Mix well, and add salt and pepper to taste. Divide the stuffing into 4 portions. Spread each cube steak with its portion and roll the steaks over the stuffing, securing with toothpicks. If it seems more convenient, you can tie rolls with string, which can be removed before serving. Place the stuffed steaks in a baking dish, add the remaining cup of bouillon, and bake for about 55 minutes, basting several times. Move the steaks to a serving platter, and either cook down or slightly thicken the baking juices with a little cornstarch. Pour this sauce over the steaks, or serve it separately.

Serves 4

TOTALS	PER RECIPE	PER SERVING
Calories	1227	307
Blocked Starch Calories	170	41
Remaining Non-Starch Calories	1057	266

BAKED FISH STEW

INGREDIENTS	CALORIES	BLOCKED STARCH CALORIES	REMAINING NON-STARCH CALORIES
Vegetable oil spray, for dish	0	0	0
1 pound white fish fillets (perch, cod, or haddock)	352	0	352
1 large onion, sliced	35	3	32
4 potatoes, sliced	480	360	120
1 cup sliced celery	20	6	14
1 tablespoon lemon juice	0	0	0
2 tablespoons tapioca	40	30	10
Salt and freshly ground pepper	0	0	0

Preheat the oven to 275°F. Spray a casserole dish with oil. Layer the fillets, onion, potatoes, and celery (in that order) in the dish. Mix the remaining ingredients with 1 cup water, and pour over the fish. Cover and bake about 2 hours.

Serves 6

TOTALS	PER RECIPE	PER SERVING
Calories	927	155
Blocked Starch Calories	399	67
Remaining Non-Starch Calories	528	88

TUNA NOODLE CASSEROLE

INGREDIENTS	CALORIES	BLOCKED STARCH CALORIES	REMAINING NON-STARCH CALORIES
1 six- or seven-ounce package noodles	612	459	153
1 can water-packed solid albacore tuna	230	0	230
½ cup sliced mushrooms	40	0	40
1 tablespoon minced onions	8	0	8
1 can cream of chicken soup	95	0	95
½ cup whole milk	75	0	75
1 teaspoon curry powder	0	0	0
Salt and freshly ground pepper	0	0	0
Vegetable oil spray, for dish	0	0	0

Preheat the oven to 350°F. Cook the noodles according to package instructions, and drain. Mix all of the ingredients and place in oiled casserole dish. Bake for about 40 minutes.

Serves 6

Totals	Per Recipe	Per Serving
Calories	1060	177
Blocked Starch Calories	459	77
Remaining Non-Starch Calories	601	100

CREAMED CHICKEN AND ASPARAGUS

Ingredients	Calories	Blocked Starch Calories	Remaining Non-Starch Calories
20 asparagus stalks	66	0	66
½ cup sliced mushrooms	20	0	20
4 slices whole wheat bread	432	324	108
4 slices roasted chicken, 3 ounces each	480	0	480
1 recipe low-calorie white sauce (see following recipe)	171	38	133
Freshly ground pepper	0	0	0

Steam the asparagus and mushrooms until tender. Toast the bread. Place 1 slice of chicken and 5 asparagus spears on each slice of toast. Mix the mushrooms and the white sauce in a saucepan and heat until boiling, stirring constantly. Pour the mushroom sauce over the asparagus, chicken, and toast. Sprinkle with black pepper.

Serves 4

Totals	Per Recipe	Per Serving
Calories	1169	292
Blocked Starch Calories	362	90
Remaining Non-Starch Calories	807	202

LOW-CALORIE STARCH-BLOCKER WHITE SAUCE

1 cup 2% milk	121	0	121
2 tablespoons all-purpose flour	50	38	12
Butter-flavored salt	0	0	0
Freshly ground pepper	0	0	0

Use about 3 tablespoons of the milk to make a thick paste with the flour. Heat the remainder of the milk to a low simmer in a small saucepan. Add the flour paste slowly, stirring constantly. Season to taste with butter-flavored salt and a touch of pepper, if desired.

Serves 4

TOTALS	PER RECIPE
Calories	171
Blocked Starch Calories	38
Remaining Non-Starch Calories	133

SHRIMP CHOW MEIN

INGREDIENTS	CALORIES	BLOCKED STARCH CALORIES	REMAINING NON-STARCH CALORIES
2 cups shrimp, cleaned and cooked	360	0	360
1 cup chopped onion	54	4	50
1 cup sliced celery	20	6	14
1 cup pea pods	145	109	36
1 cup chopped green pepper	16	0	16
1 can cream of mushroom soup	130	0	130
1 tablespoon cornstarch	30	23	7
¼ cup soy sauce	32	0	32

½ cup sliced mushrooms	40	0	40
½ cup sliced water chestnuts	40	0	40
4 cups cooked rice	800	600	200

Cook the onions, celery, pea pods, and green pepper in about 1 cup of water in a saucepan for 10 minutes. Drain, and pour back into a saucepan. Add the soup, and bring the mixture to a boil. Blend the cornstarch and soy sauce in a small bowl and add to the soup and vegetables. When the mixture is thickened, add the shrimp, mushrooms, and water chestnuts. Serve over rice.

Serves 8

TOTALS	PER RECIPE	PER SERVING
Calories	1667	208
Blocked Starch Calories	742	93
Remaining Non-Starch Calories	925	115

VEGETABLE BURGER BAKE

INGREDIENTS	CALORIES	BLOCKED STARCH CALORIES	REMAINING NON-STARCH CALORIES
2 cups pinto beans	420	315	105
1 cup fresh sprouts (bean or wheat)	30	0	30
1 small onion, diced	27	2	25
1 teaspoon hot salsa	0	0	0
2 tablespoons all-purpose flour	50	38	12
1 egg, slightly beaten	75	0	75
Salt	0	0	0

Preheat the oven to 350°F. Cook the pinto beans and mash them. Mix all the ingredients well and spread in nonstick baking dish. Bake for about 30 minutes. Cut into squares and serve hot.

Serves 6

TOTALS	PER RECIPE	PER SERVING
Calories	602	100
Blocked Starch Calories	355	59
Remaining Non-Starch Calories	247	41

BAKED CHICKEN STEW

INGREDIENTS	CALORIES	BLOCKED STARCH CALORIES	REMAINING NON-STARCH CALORIES
2 boneless, skinless chicken breasts, split	960	0	960
1 cup diced potatoes	360	270	90
1 green bell pepper, chopped	16	0	16
1 onion, chopped	35	3	32
1 cup sliced carrots	70	6	64
1 cup sliced celery	20	6	14
6 tomatoes, chopped	150	0	150
3 tablespoons instant tapioca	63	47	16
Salt and freshly ground pepper	0	0	0

Place all the ingredients in a large casserole dish with a cover, or in a crock pot. If baked in the oven, bake for 5 to 6 hours. If baked in a crock pot, follow directions.

Serves 4

TOTALS	PER RECIPE	PER SERVING
Calories	1674	419
Blocked Starch Calories	332	83
Remaining Non-Starch Calories	1342	336

RESOURCES FOR READERS

PREFERRED BRANDS OF STARCH BLOCKERS

To our knowledge, at the time of publication of this book, only Phaseolamin 2250, also called Phase 2, has been clinically tested for safety and efficacy for weight loss in humans. Therefore we only recommend brands containing Phaseolamin 2250 or Phase 2. Check for this designation on the label. If your local pharmacy, grocery store, or health food store does not carry one of the brands, refer them to www.phase2info.com for ordering information.

LOW-CARBOHYDRATE FOODS

Several major companies sell food items that have been redesigned, through ingredient substitution, to contain minimal carbohydrates, including both starch and sugar. These products are especially tailored to people with diabetes, but are also popular among people who avoid carbs for purposes of weight management. These low-carb or noncarb foods include a wide array of food items that are normally high in carbs, such as cereals, breads, cookies, candy, protein shakes, cheesecake, condiments, muffin and pancake mixes, fruit spreads, cocoa mix, ice cream, syrup, and pudding. Many of the products are very tasty and satisfying.

Following are three of the firms that provide these foods. The first, Life Services Supplements, Inc., ships foods to all locations, and has a long-standing reputation for high quality and good service. Contact them for a free catalog.

Life Services Supplements, Inc.
3535 Highway 66
Neptune, NJ 07753
800-542-3230
http://www.lifeservices.com

Carbolite Foods, Inc.
1325 Newton Avenue
Evansville, IN 47715
www.carbolitedirect.com
812-485-0002

Atkins Nutritionals, Inc.
Ronkonkoma, NY 11779
800-ATKINS

LABORATORIES THAT TEST FOR FOOD REACTIONS

A number of labs test for food reactions, including food allergies and food sensitivities. To take one of these tests, consumers have their own doctors draw blood samples, and then ship the samples to appropriate laboratories. Following are three labs that specialize in this. Contact them to determine their exact shipping procedures.

Great Smokies Diagnostic
Laboratory
63 Zillicoa Street
Asheville, NC 28801
800-522-4762

Allergy Testing Laboratory
908 NW 57th Street, Suite G
Gainesville, FL 31605
800-247-2781

Immuno Labs, Inc.
1620 West Oakland Park Blvd., Suite 300
Fort Lauderdale, FL 33311
800-231-9197

WEBSITES FOR STARCH BLOCKER INFORMATION

www.starchstopper.com
www.quantumhealth.com
Email address of Cameron Stauth: stauth@teleport.com
Email address of Steven Rosenblatt, M.D.: srosenblatt@sierramed.com

APPENDIX B

CHAPTER NOTES

Chapter One

Atkins, R.C. *Dr. Atkins' Diet Revolution*, New York: Bantam, 1972.

Brand-Miller, Jennie; Wolever, Thomas; Celagiuri, Stephen; Foster-Powell, Kaye. *The Glucose Revolution*, New York: Marlowe & Company, 1999.

Brunzell, J.D.; Austin, M.A. "Plasma triglyceride levels and coronary artery disease." *New England Journal of Medicine*, No. 320, 1989.

Challem, Jack; Berkson, Burt; Smith, Diane. *Syndrome X*, New York: John Wiley & Sons, 2001.

Gittleman, Ann Louise. *Beyond Pritikin*, Bantam, 1988.

Heller, Richard; Heller, Rachael; Vagnini, Frederic. *The Carbohydrate Addict's Healthy Heart Program*, New York: Ballantine, 1999.

Kataoka, K.; DiMagno, E.P.; Mayo Clinic. "Effect of prolonged intraluminal alpha-amylase inhibition on eating, weight, and the small intestine of rats." *Nutrition*, Vol. 15, No. 2, 1999.

Mokdad, A.H., et al., "The spread of the obesity epidemic in the United States, 1991–1998." *Journal of the American Medical Association*, No. 282, 1999.

Nathan, D.M. "Initial management of glycemia in type 2 diabetes mellitus." *New England Journal of Medicine*, No. 347, 2002.

Neergaard, L. "Federal officials opt for a new review of ephedra." The Associated Press, *The Oregonian*, June 15, 2002.

Ornish, Dean. *Dr. Dean Ornish's Program for Reversing Heart Disease*, New York: Ballantine Publishing Group, 1990.

Polivy, J., et al. "Food restriction and binge eating: A study of former prisoners of war." *Journal of Abnormal Psychology*, Vol. 103, No. 2, 1994.

Pope, Jamie. *The Last Five Pounds*, New York: Pocket Books, 1995.

Pritikin, Nathan. *The Pritikin Permanent Weight-Loss Manual*, New York: Grosset & Dunlap, 1981.

Rubino, F., et al. "Weight loss and plasma ghrelin levels." *New England Journal of Medicine*, No. 347, 2002.

Sears, Barry. *The Anti-Aging Zone*, New York: ReganBooks, 1999.

Sears, Barry. *Enter the Zone*, New York: ReganBooks, 1995.

Tappenden, K.A.; Martin, A.; Layman, Donald; Baum, J.I. "Evaluation of the efficacy of an amylase inhibitor." *FASEB Journal*, Vol. 15, No. 4, 2001.

Taubes, G. "Low-carb diet can't be dismissed." *New York Times* Syndicate, July 23, 2002.

Thom, E.; "A randomized, double-blind, placebo-controlled trial of a new weight reducing agent of natural origin." *Journal of International Medical Research,* Vol. 28, 2000.

Chapter Two

Atkins, R.C. *Dr. Atkins New Diet Revolution,* New York: M. Evans, 1992.

Choudhury, A., et al. "Character of a wheat amylase inhibitor preparation and effects on fasting human pancreatiobiliary secretions and hormones." *Gastroenterology,* Vol. 3. No. 5, 1996.

D'Adamo, P.H.; Whitney, Catherine. *Eat Right 4 Your Type,* New York: G.P. Putnam's Sons, 1996.

Eades, M.; Eades, M. *Protein Power,* New York: Bantam Books, 1996.

Eades, M. *Thin So Fast,* Warner Books, 1989.

Eaton, S.B., et al. "Stone agers in the fast lane: chronic degenerative diseases in evolutionary perspective." *American Journal of Medicine,* Vol. 8, No. 4, 1998.

Goran, M.I., et al. "Impaired glucose intolerance in obese children and adolescents." *New England Journal of Medicine,* No. 347, 2002.

Grimes, William. "Self-Denial Takes a Holiday." *The New York Times,* Nov. 26, 1997.

Hayflick, L. *How and Why We Age,* New York: Ballantine Publishing Group, 1994.

Heller, Richard; Heller, Rachael. *The Carbohydrate Addict's Diet,* Penguin, 1991.

Heller, R.F. "Hyperinsulinemic obesity and carbohydrate addiction: The missing link is carbohydrate frequency." *Medical Hypothesis,* Vol. 42, 1994.

Kannel, W.B.; Wilson, P.W.; Zhang, T.J. "The epidemiology of impaired glucose tolerance and hypertension." *American Heart Journal,* Vol. 121, No. 4, 1991.

Layer, P.; Carlson, G.L.; and DiMagno, E.P.; Mayo Clinic. "Partially purified white bean amylase inhibitor reduces starch digestion in vitro and inactivates intraduodenal amylase in humans." *Gastroenterology,* Vol. 12, 1984.

Udani, J.; Northridge Hospital, an affiliate of the University of California at Los Angeles. "Investigation of the efficacy of Phase 2 starch blockers." Publication pending, 2002.

Chapter Three

The primary sources of material for this chapter were the 45 studies that are listed in Appendix C.

Chapter Four

Allred, T.B. "Too much of a good thing? An overemphasis on eating low-fat foods may be contributing to the alarming increase in overweight among adults." *Journal of the American Dietetic Association*, Vol. 95, 1995.

The CDC Diabetes Cost Effectiveness Group. "Cost effectiveness of intensive glycemic control, intensified hypertension control, and serum cholesterol reduction for type 2 diabetes." *Journal of the American Medical Association*, No. 287, 2002.

Clouatre, Dallas. *Anti-Fat Nutrients*, San Francisco: Pax Publishing, 1997.

Eaton, S.B., et al. "Paleolithic nutrition revisited: a 12-year retrospective on its nature and implications." *European Journal of Clinical Nutrition*, Vol. 51, 1997.

Erdmann, Robert, and Jones, Meririon. *Fats That Can Save Your Life*, Encinitas, CA: Progressive Health Publishing, 1995.

Haas, Elson; Stauth, Cameron. *The False Fat Diet*, Ballantine, 2000.

Katahn, Martin. *The T-Factor Diet*, Bantam Books, 1994.

Kelley, William Donald. *The Metabolic Types*, The Kelley Foundation, 1976.

Khalsa, D.S., and Stauth, Cameron. *Brain Longevity*, New York: Warner Books, 1997.

Ludwig, D.S. "Dietary fiber, weight gain, and cardiovascular disease risk factors in young adults." *Journal of the American Medical Association*, No. 282, 1999.

McDowell, M. "Appetite control: An addiction-like component in overeating, and its cure." *Obesity and Bariatric Medicine*, No. 9, 1980.

Murray, Michael. *Hypoglycemia and Diabetes*, Rocklin, CA: Prima Publishing, 1994.

Ross, Julia. *The Diet Cure*, New York: Viking, 1999.

Royal, Fuller F. "Food allergy addiction in a bariatric practice." *Obesity and Bariatric Medicine*, Vol. 7, No. 45, 1978.

Simontacchi, Carol. *Your Fat Is Not Your Fault*, New York: Jeremy Tarcher/Putnam, 1997.

Stagnaro, S., et al. "Diet and risk of type 2 diabetes." *New England Journal of Medicine*, No. 346, 2002.

Stauth, Cameron. *The New Approach to Cancer*, New York: T.S. Vernon & Sons, 1981.

Steelman, M., et al. "Pharmacotherapy for obesity." *New England Journal of Medicine*, No. 346, 2002.

Steward, H.L.; Bethea, M.C.; Andrews, S.S.; Balart, L.A. *Sugar Busters*, New York: Ballantine Publishing Group, 1998.

Teff, K., et al. "Sweet taste: effect on dephalic phase insulin release in men." *Physiology and Behavior*, Vol. 57, No. 6, 1995.

Wolever, T.M., et al., "Metabolic response to test meals containing different carbohydrate foods: Relationship between rate of digestion and plasma insulin response." *Nutrition Research,* Vol. 8, 1988.

Wolcott, William, with Trish Fahey, *The Metabolic Typing Diet,* New York: Doubleday, 2000.

Chapter Five

Bjorntorp, P. "Thrifty genes and human obesity—are we chasing ghosts?" *Lancet,* Vol. 358, No. 1006.

Brewerton, Tim. "Toward a unified theory of serotonin dysregulation in eating and related disorders." *Psychoneuroendocrinology,* No. 6, 1955.

Christensen, L. "The roles of caffeine and sugar in depression." *Nutrition Report,* Vol. 9, No. 3.

Curzon, G. "Serotonin and appetite." *Annals of the New York Academy of Sciences,* No. 60, 1990.

Dalton, Katharina. *Once a Month,* Alameda, CA: Hunter House, 1979.

Davies, M.J., et al. "Effects of moderate alcohol intake on fasting insulin and glucose concentrations and insulin sensitivity in postmenopausal women." *Journal of the American Medical Association,* No. 287, 2002.

Des Maisons, Kathleen. *Potatoes Not Prozac,* New York: Simon and Schuster, 1998.

Des Maisons, Kathleen. *The Sugar Addict's Total Recovery Program,* New York: Ballantine Books, 2000.

Drewnowski, A.; Holden-Wiltse, J. "Changes in mood after carbohydrate consumption." *American Journal of Clinical Nutrition,* No. 46, 1987.

Fernstrom, J.D., et al. "Brain serotonin: Increase following ingestion of carbohydrate diet." *Science,* Dec. 3, 1971.

Fernstrom, J.D. "Tryptophan, serotonin and carbohydrate appetite: Will the real carbohydrate craver please stand up!" *Journal of Nutrition,* No., 118, 1988.

Forsander, D.A. "Is carbohydrate metabolism genetically related to alcohol drinking?" *Alcohol,* Vol. 1, No. 1, 1987.

Gianninni, A., et al. "Symptoms of premenstrual syndrome as a beta-endorphin: two subtypes." *Program of Neuropsychopharmacologic Biology and Psychiatry,* Vol. 18, No. 2, 1994.

Gittleman, Ann Louise. *Super Nutrition for Women,* New York: Bantam, 1991.

Hart, Carol. *Secrets of Serotonin,* New York: St. Martin's, 1996.

Helmstetter, Shad, and Schwartz, Bob. *Self-Talk for Weight Loss,* New York: St. Martin's/River Productions, 1994.

Khalsa, D.S., and Stauth, Cameron. *The Pain Cure,* New York: Warner Books, 1999.

Maccarone, D. "A well-fed family." *Psychology Today,* Oct. 2002.

Raloff, J. "How the brain knows when to stop eating." *Science News,* No. 150, 1996.

Chapter Six

Bailey, Covert. *Fit or Fat,* Boston: Houghton Mifflin, 1977.

Balady, G.J. "Survival of the fittest—more evidence." *New England Journal of Medicine,* No. 346, 2002.

Benson, S.E.; Englebert-Fenton, K.A. "Nutritional aspects of amenorrhea in the female athlete triad." *International Journal of Sports Nutrition,* No. 6, 1996.

Bernstein, L., et al. "Physical exercise and reduced risk of breast cancer in young women." *Journal of the National Cancer Institute,* No. 86, 1994.

Fiberg, R., et al. "Training down regulates fatty acid synthase in obese Zucker rats." *Medicine and Science in Sports and Exercise,* Vol. 34, No. 17, 2002.

Folson, A.R., et al. "Increase in fasting insulin and glucose over seven years with increasing weight and inactivity of young adults." *American Journal of Epidemiology,* Vol. 144, 1996.

Galbo, H.J., et al. "Glucagon and plasma catecholamine response to graded and prolonged exercise in man." *Journal of Applied Physiology,* Vol. 38, 1975.

Garcia, Oz. *The Balance,* New York: ReganBooks, 1998.

Jakicic, J.M., et al. "Effects of intermittent exercise and use of home exercise equipment on adherence, weight loss, and fitness in overweight women—a randomized trial." *Journal of the American Medical Association,* No. 282, 1999.

Hartz, D. "More children struggle with too much weight." Knight Ridder News Service, *The Oregonian,* Oct. 1, 2002.

Kraus, W. E. "Effects of the amount and intensity of exercise on plasma lipoproteins," *New England Journal of Medicine,* No. 347, 2002.

Manetta, J., et al. "Fuel oxidation during exercise in middle-aged men: role of training and glucose disposal." *Medicine and Science in Sports and Exercise,* Vol. 34, No. 3, 2002.

Paffenberger, R., et al. "Physical activity, all-cause mortality and longevity of college alumni." *New England Journal of Medicine,* No. 314, 1986.

Parr, R. B. "Exercising when you're overweight: getting in shape and shedding pounds." *The Physician and Sportsmedicine,* Vol. 24, No. 10, 1996.

Phillips, Bill. *Body for Life,* New York: HarperCollins, 2002.

Van-Dale, et al. "Does exercise give an additional effect in weight reduction regimens?" *International Journal of Obesity,* No. 11, 1987.

Chapter Seven

The sources of the material in this chapter were the patient files of Steven Rosenblatt, M.D., and interviews of patients by Steven Rosenblatt and Cameron Stauth.

Chapter Eight

American Council on Exercise. *Personal Trainer Manual for Fitness Instructors,* Boston, MA: Reebok University Press, 1991.

Asp, N. "Classification and methodology of food carbohydrates as related to nutritional effects." *American Journal of Clinical Nutrition,* No. 61, 1995.

Brand, M.J. "Importance of glycemic index in diabetes." *American Journal of Clinical Nutrition,* No. 59, 1994.

Clifford, Carey. http://www.efit.com/servlet/article/17124.html; 2002.

Crittenden, R.G., et al. "Production, properties and application of food grade oligosaccharides." *Trends in Food Science Technology,* Vol. 7, No. 353, 1997.

Gilbert, Sue. http://www.ivillage.com/food/experts/nutrition/articles/0,11731, 165839–3885,00.html; 2002.

Howley, Edward; Franks, Don. *Health Fitness Instructor's Handbook,* Second Edition, Champaign, IL: Human Kinetics, 1992.

Jenkins, D., et al. "Glycemic index of foods: a physiological basis for carbohydrate exchange." *American Journal of Clinical Nutrition,* No. 34, 1981.

Lahmayer, Ruth. "How low should calories go?" *IDEA Today,* Sept. 1989.

Pierson, Vicki. http://www.primus/web.com/fitnesspartner/library/weight/cals-burned.htm; 2002.

Prevention Magazine Editors. *Food and Nutrition,* Prevention Total Health System Series, 1984.

Roberfroid, M.; Slavin, J. "Nondigestible oligosaccharides." *Critical Reviews in Food Science and Nutrition,* Vol. 40, No. 6, 2000.

Rosenbaum, Michael; Bosco, Dominick. *Super Fitness Beyond Vitamins,* New York: Signet Books, 1989.

Truswell, A. "Glycemic index of foods." *European Journal of Clinical Nutrition,* No. 46, 1992.

Various restaurant chains, including McDonald's, Wendy's, Burger King, Jack in the Box, KFC, Taco Bell, and Arby's.

Wittenberg, Margaret M. *Good Food—The Comprehensive Food and Nutrition Resource,* Freedom, CA: The Crossing Press, 1995.

Winick, Myron. *Nutrition in Health and Disease,* Melbourne, FL: Robert E. Krieger Publishing, 1986.

Whitney, Eleanor; Cataldo, Corinne; and Rolfes, Sharon. *Understanding Normal and Clinical Nutrition,* St. Paul, MN: West Publishing Co., 1991.

Chapter Nine

Menu plans were compiled by the authors, with the assistance of Chris Ade.

Chapter Ten

The sources of the recipes were the computer files of Philippe Boulot, of the Heathman Restaurant, Portland, Oregon, and the files of Lorraine Stauth, former host of the program *Ladies First.*

APPENDIX C

DETAILS ON STUDIES

Following are citations and descriptions of the most important studies concerning starch calorie neutralization.

1970s

(1) DiMagno, E.P., et al.; Mayo Clinic, "Relations between pancreatic enzyme outputs and malabsorption in severe pancreatic insufficiency." *New England Journal of Medicine*, No. 288, 1973.

(2) Marshall, J.J.; and Lauda, C.M., "Purification and properties of phaseolamin, an inhibitor of alpha-amylase, from the kidney bean, phaseolus vulgaris." *Journal of Biological Chemistry*, No. 250, 1975. (This was one of the earliest papers to propose the concept of starch blockers.)

1981

(3) Anderson, I.A., et al., "Incomplete absorption of the carbohydrate in all-purpose wheat flour." *New England Journal of Medicine*, No. 304, 1981.

1983

(4) Hollenbeck, C.B., et al., "Effects of a commercial starch blocker preparation on carbohydrate metabolism and absorption in vivo and in vitro studies." *American Journal of Clinical Nutrition*, No. 38, 1983.

(5) Carlson, G.E., et al., "A bean a-amylase inhibitor formulation (starch blocker) is ineffective in man." *Science*, No. 219, 1983. (This noted the failure of early, crude ground-bean preparations to inhibit starch digestion.)

1984

(6) Layer, P.; Carlson, G.L.; and DiMagno, E.P.; Mayo Clinic, "Partially purified white bean amylase inhibitor reduces starch digestion in vitro and inactivates intraduodenal amylase in humans." *Gastroenterology*, Vol. 12,

1984. (This was the first major, documented success using a new, purified, concentrated formula. Authors concluded that the formula "decreased in vitro digestion of dietary starch in a dose-dependent manner.")

1987

(7) Boivin, M.; Zinmesister, A.R.; Vay, L.W.; and DiMagno, E.P.; Mayo Clinic, "Effect of a purified amylase inhibitor on carbohydrate metabolism after a mixed meal in healthy humans." *Mayo Clinic Proceedings,* Vol. 62, 1987. (This was one of the early studies that explored the possibility of using starch blockers against diabetes.)

1989

(8) Jain, N.K., et al.; Mayo Clinic, "Effect of ileal perfusion of carbohydrates and amylase inhibitor on gastrointestinal hormones and emptying." *Gastroenterology,* Vol. 16, 1989.

1991

(9) Yamaguchi, H., "Isolation and characterization of the subunits of phaseolus vulgaris alpha amylase inhibitor." *Journal of Biochemistry,* Vol. 110, No. 5, 1991. (This was the first Japanese study. In it, two subunits of amylase inhibitors were discovered in white kidney beans.)

1992

(10) Yamadera, K.; Sandberg, R.J.; and DiMagno, E.P.; Mayo Clinic, "Can chronic ingestion of a wheat amylase inhibitor (AI) reduce insulin secretion without producing malabsorption in dogs?" *Pancreas,* Vol. 7, No. 6, p. 762, 1992.

(11) Yamadera, K., et al.; Mayo Clinic, "Can wheat amylase inhibitors (AI) lower pancreatic amylase activity sufficiently to cause carbohydrate malabsorption?" *Gastroenterology,* Vol. 102, No. 4, 1992.

(12) Umoren, J.; and Kies, C.; Northern Illinois University, "Commercial soybean starch blocker consumption: impact on weight gain and on copper, lead, and zinc status of rats." *Plant Foods in Human Nutrition,* Vol. 42, No. 2, 1992.

(13) Yamashita, H., et al.; Kyoto University, "Inhibition and binding modes of low molecular weight inhibitors of porcine pancreatic alpha-amylase." *Journal of Biochemistry,* Vol. 3, No. 2, 1992.

1994

(14) Pueyo, J.J., et al.; University of California, San Diego, "Activation of bean phaseolus vulgaris alpha-amylase inhibitor requires proteolytic processing of the proprotein." *Plant Physiology,* Vol. 101, No. 4, 1993.

(15) Yamaguchi, H.; Kyoto University, "Isolation and characterization of the subunits of a heat-labile alpha-amylase inhibitor from phaseolus vulgaris white kidney bean." *Biosci Biotechnology and Biochemistry,* Vol. 57, No. 2, 1993. (This study and the following study were continuations of the effort to concentrate and purify an amylase inhibitor.)

(16) Furuichi, Y., et al.; Mie University, "Some characteristics of an alpha-amylase inhibitor from phaseolus vulgaris (cultivar great northern) seeds." *Biosci Biotechnology and Biochemistry,* Vol. 57, No. 1, 1993.

(17) Suetsuna, K., et al.; Shimonoseki University, "Structure of an alpha-amylase inhibitor produced by marine actinomycete and its lowering effects in vivo of glucose and lipid in blood." *Journal of Shimonoseki University of Fisheries,* Vol. 42, No. 4, 1994. (This was one of the early studies indicating that starch blockers suppressed insulin elevation in diabetic animals.)

1995

(18) Doi, T., et al.; Kyushu University, "Alpha-amylase inhibitor increases plasma 3-hydroxybutyric acid in food restricted rats." *Experientia,* Vol. 51, No. 6, 1995. (This was the first indirect indication that use of starch blockers may partially inhibit development of colon cancer cells.)

(19) Koike, D.; Yamadera, K.; and DiMagno, E.P.; Mayo Clinic, "Effect of a wheat amylase inhibitor on canine carbohydrate digestion, gastrointestinal function, and pancreatic growth." *Gastroenterology,* Vol. 108, No. 4, 1995. (This Mayo Clinic study investigated starch blockers for weight loss.)

(20) Choudhury, A.; and DiMagno, E.P.; Mayo Clinic, "Does a wheat amylase inhibitor (WAI) affect intraduodenal amylase activity in humans?" *Gastroenterology,* Vol. 108, No. 4, 1995. (This was another of the continuing series of Mayo Clinic investigations into the use of starch blockers for diabetes.)

1996

(21) Choudhury, A., et al.; Mayo Clinic, "Character of a wheat amylase inhibitor preparation and effects on fasting human pancreatiobiliary

secretions and hormones." *Gastroenterology,* Vol. 3, No. 5, 1996. (This study noted that "amylase inhibition induces carbohydrate tolerance, satiety, and weight loss, and prolongs gastric emptying, effects that may be useful in the treatment of obesity and diabetes mellitus.")

(22) Finardi-Filho, F., et al.; U. of California, San Diego, "A putative precursor protein in the evolution of the bean alpha-amylase inhibitor." *Phytochemistry,* Vol. 43, No. 1, 1996.

1997

(23) LeBerre-Anton, V., et al.; Toulouse Cedex, "Characterization and functional properties of the alpha-amylase inhibitor from kidney bean seeds." *Biochimica et Biophysica Acta,* Vol. 134, No. 1, 1997. (This study indicated the lack of toxic effects of starch blockers.)

(24) Lankisch, M.R.; Lager, P.; and DiMagno, E.P.; Mayo Clinic, "Does prandial intake of a wheat amylase inhibitor (WAI) affect hormones that regulate carbohydrate metabolism or gut function in normal, obese, or diabetic persons?" *Gastroenterology,* Vol. 112, No. 4, 1997.

(25) Nakaguchi, T., et al.; Osaka University, "Structural characterization of an alpha-amylase inhibitor from a wild common bean: insight into the common structural features of leguminous alpha-amylase inhibitors." *Journal of Biochemistry,* Vol. 121, No. 2, 1997.

1998

(26) Ihara, K., et al.; Kyushu University, "Prevention of hypoglycemia in a patient with type Ib glycogen storage disease by an amylase (alpha-glucosidase) inhibitor." *Acta Paediatrica,* Vol. 87, No. 5.

(27) Lankisch, M.; Layer, P.; Rizza, R.A.; DiMagno, E.P.; Mayo Clinic, "Acute postprandial gastrointestinal and metabolic effects of wheat amylase inhibitor (WAI) in normal, obese, and diabetic humans." *Pancreas,* Vol. 17, No. 2., 1998.

(28) Kataoka, K.; DiMagno, E.P.; Mayo Clinic, "Effect of chronic amylase inhibition on pancreatic growth and acinar cell secretory function in rats." *Pancreas,* Vol. 17, No. 2, 1998.

(29) Feick, P., et al.; University of Saarland, Germany, "Pervanadate stimulates amylase release and protein tyrosine phosphorylation of paxillin and p125(FAK) in differentiated AR4–2J pancreatic acinar cells." *Journal of Biological Chemistry,* Vol. 273, No. 26, 1998.

1999

(30) Young, N.M., et al.; National Research Council of Canada, "Post-translational processing of two alpha-amylase inhibitors and an arcelia from the common bean, phaseolus vulgaris." *F.E.B.S. Letters,* Vol. 446, No. 1, 1999.

(31) Kataoka, K.; DiMagno, E.P.; Mayo Clinic, "Effect of prolonged intraluminal alpha-amylase inhibition on eating, weight, and the small intestine of rats." *Nutrition,* Vol. 15, No. 2, 1999. (In this study, rats fed a starch inhibitor gained less weight than a control group of rats.)

(32) Yoshikawa, H., et al., "Characterization of kintoki bean (phaseolus vulgaris) alpha-amylase inhibitor: inhibitory activities against human salivary and porcine pancreatic alpha-amylases and activity changes by proteolytic digestion." *Journal of Nutritional Science,* Vol. 45, No. 6, 1997. (This was one of the long series of Japanese experiments aimed at increasing the potency of starch blockers.)

2000

(33) Iulek, J., et al.; University of Ponta Grossa, Brazil, "Purification, biochemical characterization and partial primary structure of new alpha-amylase inhibitor from Secale cereal (rye)." *International Journal of Biochemistry and Cell Biology,* Vol. 32, No. 11–12, 2000.

(34) Wato, S., et al.; Osaka University, "A chimera-like alpha-amylase inhibitor suggesting the evolution of phaseolus vulgaris alpha-amylase inhibitor." *Journal of Biochemistry,* Vol. 128, No. 1, 2000.

(35) Thom, E.; "A randomized, double-blind, placebo-controlled trial of a new weight reducing agent of natural origin." *Journal of International Medical Research,* Vol. 28, 2000. (In this 12-week study of 40 obese volunteers, people using starch blockers lost an average of 3.5 kg., compared to an average of 1.2 kg. lost by a control group. Eighty-five percent of the lost weight was adipose tissue.)

2001

(36) Tappenden, K.A.; Martin, A.; Layman, Donald; and Baum, J.I.; University of Illinois, "Evaluation of the efficacy of an amylase inhibitor;" *FASEB Journal,* Vol. 15, No. 4, 2001. (Researchers determined that a starch blocker decreased amylase activity by 50% to 75%, and remarked that this outcome "supports the hypothesis that an amylase inhibitor may reduce or delay carbohydrate digestion and glucose absorption.")

(37) Hansawasdi, C., et al.; Hokkaidō University, "Hibiscus acid as an inhibitor

of starch digestion in the Caco-2 cell model system." *Biosci Biotechnology and Biochemistry,* Vol. 65, 2001. (This study indicated that the hibiscus plant contains starch blockers, but that the concentration is not sufficient for use in humans.)

(38) Douglas, D.J., et al.; University of British Columbia, "Detection of noncovalent complex between alpha-amylase and its microbial inhibitor tendamistat by electrospray ionization mass spectrometry." *Rapid Communication Mass Spectrometry,* Vol. 15, 2001.

(39) Maheshwari, R., "Acute toxicity study of Phase 2 starch neutralizer." Unpublished, 2001. Details available at www.starchstopper.com. (In a series of two studies, rats were fed high dosages of the Phase 2 formulation of starch blocker, were monitored for side effects, sacrificed, and autopsied. No negative side effects occurred. The study was conducted off-premises by a researcher for the National Institutes of Health.)

(40) Vinson, J.A.; University of Scranton, "Investigation of the efficacy of Phase 2, a purified bean extract from Pharmachem Laboratories." Publication pending, 2001. Details available at www.starchstopper.com. (A group of 10 volunteers were given Phase 2 starch blockers prior to eating starchy foods, and were then monitored in regard to plasma glucose. Volunteers taking starch blockers had a plasma-glucose time curve that was an average of 57% lower than that of the control group. Researchers called the outcome "promising, positive preliminary results.")

(41) Vinson, J.A.; and Shuta, D.; University of Scranton, "In vivo effectiveness of a starch absorption blocker in a double-blind, placebo-controlled study with normal college-age subjects." Publication pending, 2001. Details available at www.starchstopper.com. (Starch digestion inhibition was found to occur at an 85% level of effectiveness among subjects taking the Phase 2 formulation of starch blockers.)

(42) Vinson, J.A.; University of Scranton, "Efficacy of Phase 2 when taken with a mixed meal." Publication pending, 2001. Details available at www.starchstopper.com (750 mg. of Phase 2 starch blocker material were mixed into a Hungry Man TV dinner, resulting in the blockage of 28% of starch calories. The results indicated that 750 mg. was not a sufficient dosage to ensure robust starch calorie neutralization).

2002

(43) Ballerini, R.; Pharmaceutical Development and Service of Italy, "Evaluation of the effectiveness of Phase 2." Publication pending, 2002. Details available at www.starchstopper.com. (Sixty volunteers, age 20 to 45, were

randomly assigned to take Phase 2 starch blocker or a placebo. Volunteers on Phase 2 lost an average of 6.45 pounds over 30 days, compared to an average weight loss of 3/4 pound among volunteers on placebo.)

(44) Sathe, Shri; University of Florida, "Additional safety study to investigate phytohemagglutinizing activity and protein malabsorption in Phase 2." Unpublished, 2002. (The experiments indicated that the Phase 2 starch blocker material has no negative effects upon protein digestion, or upon the cardiovascular system.)

(45) Udani, J.; Northridge Hospital, an affiliate of the University of California at Los Angeles, "Investigation of the efficacy of Phase 2 starch blockers." Publication pending, 2002. (In this study, presented in detail in Chapter Three, volunteers taking starch blockers achieved a combined weight loss that was 230% higher than that achieved by volunteers on placebo, while experiencing a higher level of well-being than subjects on placebo.)

INDEX